The Herbal Remedies and Natural Remedies Bible [10 in 1]

The Most Extensive Selection of Healing Herbs and Plants to Nurture for Realising Natural Antibiotics, Essential Oils, Infusions and Tinctures

By

Bruce Holmes

Contents

Introduction

People are growing increasingly interested in natural healing and wellness, which has led to a rise in the popularity of herbalism, part of the oldest & most powerful therapeutic methods. It's a go-to for common health issues and for boosting general wellness. Herbs are plants with medicinal properties. The term "natural healing" now encompasses a wide range of practices that rely on natural elements to promote health. Most herbal treatments come from plants, but others are made from minerals or even animals. Phytotherapy refers to the study of how plants may be used to cure disease. Natural elements are used to create herbal treatments, which aid the body's recuperative processes. Herbal medicines are becoming more popular as a means of maintaining health. If you're looking to maintain or enhance your general health, herbal treatments may help. Herbal treatments are often consumed as teas or diluted in Water because of this. Honey or lemon juice, for example, might be added to herbal treatments to increase their efficacy. Native American healing practices are influenced by and reflect significant cultural viewpoints. The world of herbal medicine opens up a brand-new, all-natural domain of healing to you as well as your family as you continue on your path. Regardless of your passion for herbalism, you will experience a good impact on your life. It is only one among the many lovely consequences of holistic treatment. It wasn't the intention of your therapy with that one plant or that herbal combination to make you feel better mentally, but it did. Alkaloids and flavonoids, which are often present in medicinal plants, offer powerful therapeutic properties. Every herbal medicine cabinet must include medicinal herbs. Humans have used them for centuries to cure illnesses and diseases. Your physical and emotional health may both benefit from having garden space at home. It may grow into a delightful activity that you can share with others to encourage them to lead better lifestyles.

Each herb has a unique combo of specific characteristics in addition to certain fairly wide effects on some emotional systems. By carefully matching the herbal properties of the symptoms that are being treated, it can be accomplished to address every aspect of the disease at once, which leads to a cure as rapidly to be possible and with the tiniest possible doses.

Herbal medicine has been used for a wide variety of conditions and symptoms for hundreds of years. Many different societies have used herbal treatments at various points throughout history. Herbs were important to ancient Egyptian medicine and rituals. Some old walls include hieroglyphics depicting the medicinal usage of plants. Herbal treatments make use of several plants, including those with medicinal properties. People cure their illnesses with herbal medications and also utilize them to stay healthy. They make use of them in order to alleviate symptoms, enhance energy levels, relax, or drop weight.

Herbal therapies are often quite safe when taken properly and have fewer adverse effects than conventional pharmaceuticals. Overuse of antibiotics is one way in which the body might develop resistance to the drug. Herbal remedies are effective for treating mild to moderate ailments. Herbs may be used in several therapeutic contexts. As you know, there are numerous benefits to treating your kid with natural and at-home treatments, whether they have a small illness like head lice, chicken pox, headache, or painful toothache. Whether your family lacks health insurance or your youngster just fears going to the doctor's office, think about trying a natural cure first. The outcomes could gratify both yourself and your kid.

Because a lot of the materials required for natural remedies can be obtained in most households, they are also sometimes referred to as "home remedies." As a result, treating a kid at home is simple and practical. The time and money saved must also be mentioned. Travel and expensive excursions to the pharmacy or doctor's office are eliminated with home treatments.

BOOK 1: Herbal Apothecary

The leaves, stems, bark, roots, flowers, and seeds of numerous medicinal plants are used to make herbal remedies. The usage of medicinal herbs is still quite common. Today, more than one-third of Americans utilize herbal remedies to treat a range of diseases and conditions.

1.1 What Do Apothecaries Do? Past to the Present

The word "apothecary" has an alluring and enigmatic ring to it. You may faintly see it as a store selling plants or compare it to one of the mystical stores in Harry Potter, which offered items like unicorn horns and bug eyeballs. What, however, is an apothecary exactly? Apothecaries were around for hundreds of thousands of decades, but the Middle Ages saw their greatest popularity. They finally disappeared in the nineteenth century as a result of modifications to society's institutions and medical practices. Apothecary stores still exist today, despite the fact that they have changed significantly. Apothecaries once again play a significant role in society since there is increased interest in holistic health and natural treatment methods.

What do apothecaries do?

An apothecary is what, exactly? Historically, the term "apothecary" might denote either a person who manufactured and sold medications or a store where they sold their wares, much like a pharmacy today.

House of apothecary

The term "apothecary" eventually came to be used to refer to the stores that were controlled by apothecaries and in which various goods were sold. You may consider them as the forerunners of pharmacies as we know them today. You may purchase ready-made medications from them, in addition to other items like soaps, spices, beauty products, dyes, and so on.

The majority of the items that could be purchased in these stores were from natural sources; nevertheless, the components and methods of preparation evolved with time. They provided people with access to medicinal herbs, spices, and items that they otherwise would not have had if they were responsible for the cultivation and production of all of their own food and goods.

The person who is an apothecary

The vast majority of the medications made, compounded, and dosed by apothecaries were created using herbs along with other natural materials. They served as both doctors and pharmacists in the past. People would enter their store and inform them about ailments, accidents, or imbalances.

The apothecary would proceed to formulate the patient's medication after making a diagnosis and suggestion. The majority of apothecaries obtained their training by spending several years as apprentices with an experienced apothecary. They had to acquire a variety of abilities, including accurate plant identification and harvesting, producing medical concoctions, calculating the right doses for various individuals, diagnosing illnesses, etc. It's easy to assume that apothecaries have been either scammers or unqualified for their job given the prevalence of our current medical system, yet the opposite is really true. There can never be "wrong apples" in any field, but the majority of apothecaries took satisfaction in their work and in helping people. Many spent years in the classroom learning and staying current with science and medicine. In order to maintain rigorous requirements for the quality of medicines and components offered, guilds were established in Britain and other nations. The neighborhood pharmacy used to be an important part of every community and metropolis.

1.2 Apothecary Evolution and Apothecary Decline

Evolution: Both the business and the practice of becoming an apothecary underwent various transformations and developments in function as time went on. Beginning in the 1700s, several pharmacies and other medical facilities started to include apothecary stores inside their existing structures.

1.   This marked the starting point of a transition from apothecaries serving as both physicians and pharmacists to playing a job that is more synonymous with that of a pharmacist solely.

Even while many people retained a significant amount of knowledge about fundamental therapeutic practices, their attention turned more toward the creation of high-quality medicines and the comprehension of plant and chemical ingredients. Naturally, in more rural areas where there were no hospitals or medical offices, apothecaries continued to operate in a manner somewhat unlike how they had in the past. A further transformation took place in the middle of the nineteenth century with the introduction of patented medication (including natural remedies) along with the rise of the wandering salesman. A guy called Samuel Thomson was instrumental in the development of this new movement in the United States. He devised a way of medicinal plants, patented several treatments, and did extensive travel teaching others his techniques.

2.   Although he was ultimately unsuccessful, he did usher in a novel approach to the business of marketing pharmaceuticals.

As a direct consequence of this development, the need for apothecaries has significantly decreased in recent years. People were able to purchase goods from itinerant salesmen and get medical guidance and supplies from a variety of different organizations.

Decline: Although it's possible to say that, throughout time, apothecaries went out of business nearly entirely, this statement wouldn't be completely accurate. In many communities, the apothecary as an occupation and as a business that offered natural and herbal remedies became extinct; nonetheless, it maintained a footing in certain regions so that it may emerge again in the future. On the other hand, in another way, apothecaries transformed into what we today refer to as pharmaceuticals. The use of isolated chemicals derived from plants, which were later recreated synthetically in laboratories, became more prevalent in medical practice. Because medicinal preparations were more standardized and sold in already packaged form, there wasn't any longer an assumption that there was a need for medical specialists who could create personalized dosages.

1.3 Advanced apothecaries

Even in this day and day, there are still businesses that go by the term "apothecary," however, it is somewhat more challenging to locate someone who describes themselves as an experienced apothecary. Apothecaries are once again becoming places where you may purchase herbs, loose green tea, organic items, and a variety of other goods as a result of the recent uptick in the popularity of herbal treatments and alternative medicine. Some of them have made their way online and evolved into expanded copies of the originals. Others continue to operate as smaller neighborhood businesses. The proprietors of apothecaries often have a great deal of knowledge about various plants and the effects they have, and they frequently formulate their own remedies. You may get a lot of knowledge from them, as well as suggestions for various herbs to utilize and what is associated with them (but they cannot provide you with professional advice).

BOOK 2: Salve and Tinctures Made from Herbs

At White, the town of Cypress, we utilize a variety of extra hand-made, organic products, such as salves, balms, and tinctures, in order to alleviate symptoms or boost the immune system as a whole.

2.1 Tinctures of Herbs: What Are They?

Tinctures of herbs are highly concentrated extracts of plants that may be created from either dried or fresh herbs. After being macerated in alcohol, the herbs produce an extract in liquid form that may be taken orally after being processed in this manner. Tinctures provide a hassle-free alternative to preparing teas and decoctions in order to take benefit of the various medicinal characteristics that plants possess. Tinctures made from herbs often have a shelf life of many years and are an excellent method for receiving every advantage of herbs with only a couple of drops. Because they don't require much room, they are also quite easy to transport about with you wherever you go. Tinctures made from herbs may be consumed on their own, or they can be combined with other liquids such as tea, Water, or lemonade.

As was previously noted, herbal tinctures are highly concentrated extracts that are created by soaking dried or new herbs in ethanol or glycerin in order to extract the therapeutic components of the plants. Oral administration is possible, and research suggests that they possess more therapeutic value and greater bioavailability than other types of herbal treatments. If, on the other hand, you have an intolerance to liquor or are abstaining from it for reasons that are private or religious in nature, you should think about using alternate forms of herbal medicines, such as teas, pills, or infusions, rather than alcohol.

What are the Benefits of Using Tinctures?

Digestion, the operation of the immune system, and the management of stress may all be helped by herbal medicines. Tinctures made from herbs may be beneficial to one's overall well-being and health.

Why Should You Make Use of Herbal Tinctures?

Tinctures made from herbs are popular due they offer a quick and simple method for obtaining the medicinal benefits of plants without the time and effort required to prepare herbal teas or decoctions. Tinctures have a shelf life of many years, which makes them an excellent method for extracting the most benefit from your plants. In addition, just a very tiny quantity of herbal tincture is required to get the desired effect. Additionally, they are simple to modify and tailor to the specific requirements and preferences of the user. You just need a few drops of a plant extract to get all of its positive effects. In general, herbal medicines are a straightforward and hassle-free method of reaping the full advantages offered by herbs. You may take advantage of the medicinal effects of herbs without having to prepare tea or decoctions by utilizing components of a high grade and consuming them in just a tiny quantity at a time. Before beginning any new medication or supplement, you should always be sure to contact your primary care physician first.

Which Herbs Are Most Frequently Employed?

Tinctures are extracted as liquid medications that may be manufactured from nearly any kind of plant. Herbs such as root, Chamomile, milk thistle, feverfew, ginger, and garlic, among many more, are often combined with alcohol to create tinctures. You may also get a wide variety of various kinds of herbal combinations that comprise a number of different therapeutic plants. Depending on the intended effect, tinctures produced from herbs may be prepared using either a single herb at a time or a mixture of many distinct plants.

How Much of an Effect Do Herbal Tinctures Have?

Tinctures made from herbs may be quite beneficial, provided that they are consumed in the appropriate manner. In order to derive the most advantage from the tincture, it is essential to make sure you are only working with herbs of the highest possible quality. In addition to this, it is vital to ensure that the dose recommendations on the bottle of tincture are adhered to. The efficacy of the tincture might be compromised either by taking it excessively or insufficiently of it. Before ingesting any herbal tinctures, it is advisable to discuss the appropriate dose with your healthcare professional, especially if you are unclear about what it should be. Tinctures made from herbs may be a great method to get the benefits of those plants without having to go through a lot of trouble if they are used correctly and cared for properly.

Tinctures made from herbs may be a very potent and useful method for gaining the benefits of those plants, provided that they are handled and used correctly. Tinctures made from herbs may be blended with the active ingredients of other natural medicines to provide even more potent results. For instance, mixing herbal tinctures plus aromatic oils or other herbs may assist in improving the effectiveness of both, resulting in even greater outcomes. Always get the OK from your doctor or other qualified medical professional before using any given combination of medicines.

Take into consideration the Tincture's Quality as well as its Source.

The efficacy of the herbal medicine you take might be significantly influenced, both directly and indirectly, by its quality and origin. Look for tinctures that are produced from herbs that have been cultivated in an environmentally responsible manner and that have been prepared using the most effective methods. In addition, regardless of where you make your purchase, the seller needs to provide you with comprehensive information on the potency, dose, and security of their wares.

When Should You Choose an Herbal Tincture?

Tinctures made from herbs are becoming more and more popular among those who are looking for natural health alternatives. But how can you determine whether or not they are the best option for you? Keep reading to find out more about some useful suggestions for deciding whether they are a good match for assessing if they an appropriate match for your requirements.

2.2 What exactly is a salve?

A salve is essentially any kind of calming or therapeutic concoction made from herbs, wax from bees and mixed oils. Although they are used for a variety of purposes, they have a history in herbal medicine that has been used for hundreds of thousands of years as remedies for illnesses or irritability. Salves may be made with a wide variety of organic components, which is why they are so renowned and have been utilized so often across history.

What purpose do salves serve?

In order to cure medical diseases or to offer calming comfort, salves and other products that are quite similar to them are applied to the tissues or scars. Salves are great items that have a wide range of applications that are nearly as diverse as the variety of materials that may be used to make them.

For example, several salves are applied topically to the epidermis as lip balms or skincare products to help penetrate and hydrate the skin. They will contain moisturizing components coming from organic materials such as flowers, origins, or fruits. These components will come from nature. An excellent illustration of this is aloe vera, which is widely regarded as one of the most effective naturally occurring emollients that can still be discovered in the wild. Because of this, they are fantastic to use as agents to preserve your skin throughout the harsh winter months, regardless of whether you just have inherently dry skin. There are a variety of different balms that might be utilized for safeguarding your skin. Your skin might become somewhat more robust and healthier with the use of certain organic oils, hence decreasing the likelihood that it will crack or break. The oil of coconut, oil of olives, oils with herbal infusions, oil from sweet almonds, and many more are some examples of others. There are a variety of different salves that may be used to feed and fortify your skin. In most cases, they are made using organic and natural components that are high in levels of various antioxidants and vitamins. Antioxidants are substances that may protect cells from the molecular damage caused by free radicals, while nutrients are what nearly every biological system within the body requires in order to function properly and rebuild itself. Antioxidants can be found in foods and supplements. One of the greatest natural substances that may be used in these kinds of salves is calendula, which is a sort of plant. Even beyond these applications, salves may be appreciated for the calming effect they provide. Applying a quality herbal salve to the skin may help cure a variety of skin conditions, including diaper rash, sunburn, and more. You will provide relief to an infected or irritated region of skin, such as a sunburn, diaper rash, bug bites, or insect bites, and you will also speed up the healing process of wounds. Redness, dryness, or discomfort. This is due to the fact that many of the greatest salves are manufactured with components that may calm and relax the skin, such as herbal oils, including blue Chamomile, which is one of the plants that is used the most across the whole globe.

What kinds of things do saves contain in their composition?

It is possible to make salves out of a wide variety of components, but the finest ones are often prepared from a combination of natural and organic materials. This is due to the fact that natural components are the things that remedies have been manufactured from throughout history. These ingredients give multiple advantages all at once, so there is no need to change something that is successful.

The following is a brief list of common components that may be found in high-quality salves; however, this list is in no way meant to be all-inclusive:

Arnica: A kind of flower that, due to the presence of its vital oils and lipids, is capable of providing pain relief.

Advantages of Using Arnica

- Hair loss

- Skin bruising

- Pain management

Aloe Vera: A kind of plant that is known not only for its high nutrient and antioxidant levels but also for its ability to act as a natural moisturizer.

Advantages of Aloe Vera

- Aloe Vera helps decrease dental plaque

- Aloe Vera includes antibacterial and antioxidants

- Burns might heal more rapidly when aloe vera is used

- Diabetics who use aloe vera may see a reduction in their blood sugar levels

- Laxative effects have been attributed to the use of aloe vera

- Mouth ulcers are treatable with aloe vera

- It's possible that aloe vera will make your skin seem better

- Gastric discomfort may be alleviated with aloe vera

- Rashes and irritations are two of the conditions that aloe vera may help

- It's possible that aloe vera may assist women in beating breast cancer

- Aloe vera may relieve dandruff

- There is some evidence that aloe vera may benefit cardiovascular health

- It's possible that aloe vera will help prevent cavities

Beeswax: This natural wax that is made by honeybees is intricate, and it contains many nutrients and vitamins that give a wide range of health advantages.

Advantages of Beeswax

- Moisturizes Skin

- Provides Relief from Eczema, Psoriasis, and Diaper Dermatitis

- Serves to safeguard the liver

- Reduces Pain While Also Acting as an Anti-Inflammatory

- Maintains a Healthier Cholesterol Balance

- Helps to Get Rid of Acne

- Helps Decrease Signs of Stretching

- Used to Treat Chapped and Dry Lips

- Reduces the effects of stress and encourages relaxation

- Aids in the Treatment of Jock Itch and Other Skin Infections Caused by Fungi

Calendula: This easy-to-grow plant is loaded with antioxidants that may be used in a wide range of salve formulations; in addition, it performs an excellent job of hydrating the skin and shielding it from environmental toxins.

Calendula's Many Uses and Benefits

- Reduce the risk of excessive blood clotting by acting as an anti-thrombogenic

- Anti-inflammatory medication that helps reduce inflammation

- Contribute to the battle against cancer (anticancer)

- Have a favorable impact on the levels of sugar in the blood (antidiabetic)

- Protecting the brain (effects that are neuroprotective)

Blue Chamomile: This blooming plant may calm and relax the outermost layer of skin while simultaneously toning and safeguarding the cells that make up the skin.

The advantages of blue Chamomile

- Healing of wounds, including ulcers and other sores and wounds

- Gastrointestinal distress in the form of indigestion, feeling sick, or gas

- Relaxation techniques

- Pain alleviation and anti-inflammatory properties for those suffering from illnesses such as arthritis, headaches, or back pain

- Providing relief from skin diseases such as eczema and rashes

- Fostering restful sleep

Chickweed: This blooming plant is loaded with multiple nutrients and is famous for its ability to hydrate and calm the skin. It is an ingredient used in many of the best salves.

Advantages of Chickweed

- Asthma

- Constipation

- Obesity

- Muscle and bone aches

- Psoriasis

- When administered directly to the skin, it may treat a variety of skin disorders, particularly comes to boil and ulcers.

Cocoa butter: This oil, which may be produced from cocoa beans, is rich in several nutrients, including fatty acids, nutrients, and antioxidants. It is beneficial in a number of ways, including providing sustenance, safeguarding, and miniaturization.

Advantages of using cocoa butter

- Keep Your Body's Skin Moisturized

- Get Vitamin E

- Skin Repair Properties

- Improved Cholesterol Levels That Are Healthier

- Defend Excessive Sun Radiation

- Better Condition of the Bones

Cinnamon: This plant is cultivated for its fragrant bark, which is harvested and used commercially as a flavoring agent. However, in addition to that, it has a number of vital nutrients, antioxidants, and vitamins.

The Advantages of Cinnamon

- It reduces swelling and inflammation in the body.

- It includes plant components that have antioxidant qualities that protect against damage.

- It would seem to be beneficial in protecting oneself from infection

- It could assist with managing blood sugar

- According to several studies, cinnamon may help guard against the common cold and influenza.

- It would suggest that cinnamon might assist in lowering the probability of developing insulin resistance.

- Cinnamon, when consumed on a regular basis, has the potential to lower blood pressure.

- There is some evidence that the chemicals found in cinnamon may decrease the progression of Alzheimer's disease.

- It contributes to a reduction in cholesterol levels

- Cinnamon may be able to lower blood pressure when consumed on a regular basis

- It is possible that it may assist in restoring the natural balance between bacteria in the digestive system, which will promote healthy digestive function.

Eucalyptus: These evergreen plants have a high concentration of antioxidants, aromatic compounds, and tannins, all of which are beneficial to the skin since they cleanse, calm, and refresh it.

The Advantages of Eucalyptus

- Pain relief

- High antioxidant levels

- Congestion in the nose and throat, colds, and breathing problems

- Oral health improvement

- Immunity booster

Jojoba seed oil: is an ingredient that may be found in a range of products designed for the hair and skin nowadays. Due to the fact that it has a very high concentration of antioxidants and fatty acids, it is ideal for calming, hydrating, cleaning, and rebalancing the skin.

Jojoba seed oil has Benefited.

- Extended Hydration and Soothing Effects

- Deeply-Hydrating

- Nutritious for Skin

- Soothes Dry Skin

- Non-Acnegenic

- Anti-Aging

- Easy, Not Greasy

- Calms and nourishes dry skin

- Gentle & Non-Allergenic

Ginger: The roots of this blooming plant are very rich in nutrients, including minerals, lipids, oils that are essential, and vitamins. If you apply it properly, it may give your skin a powerful boost.

The Advantages of Ginger

- Infections may be avoided with ginger

- Slows Cancer

- Bloating and gas

- Nausea relief

Lemon balm: This blossoming plant is strongly related to minty and is composed of complex components such as antioxidants, aromatic compounds, and tannins. Mint is a member of the Mint family. Because of this, it is calming, purifying, and pleasant to the body.

The Advantages of Lemon Balm

- It may be helpful in lowering anxiety

- It has the potential to alleviate stress

- It has the potential to improve cognitive performance

- It's possible that it might help alleviate cold sores

- It has the potential to alleviate symptoms of insomnia along with other sleep disorders

- It is an effective treatment for nausea

Rosehip seed oil: The kernels of wild rosebushes may be processed in a machine to produce this oil. If done properly, it has the potential to provide a number of advantages, including hydration, calming, protection, and others.

Advantages of using Rosehip seed oil

- **Acne** Relief

- Skin Protection

- **Eczema** Treatment

Myrrh: This well-known resin obtained from the Commiphora tree has the ability to calm, hydrate, and tone the skin.

The Advantages of Myrrh

- May Be Beneficial to Oral Health

- Eliminates Dangerous Bacteria

- Promotes Skin Wellness and May Assist in the Healing of Wounds

- Could Be a Very Effective Antioxidant

- Reduces Pain as well as Swelling

- It is a Killer for Some Parasites

2.3 The Explanation of Preparation of the Herbal Salve

- To begin, gather the blossoms and leaves straight from the garden. Take these plants that are showing signs of minor wilting, slice them up, and then store them loosely in a jar made of clean glass. Next, cut up about one cup of the leaves. (In this instance, roughly diced up half a cup of comfrey and half a cup of plantain leaves).

- Cover using about 1 and 1/2 cups of oil. You may use sunflower oil, olive oil, or sesame oil in its place. Alternatively, you may often use a mixture of grapeseed oil and coconut oil. Because our predecessors did not have the luxury of using pressed oils, they created their own medicinal ointments out of animal fats such as lard, bear oil, and other animal-based oils, all of which are said to have their own inherent healing properties.

- A strip of cheesecloth or a filter for coffee that has been attached with an elastic band should be used to cover the entire top of the jar. Because of this, moisture in the jar that would have otherwise spoiled the salve is able to escape.

- The next step is to place the jar on a sunny ledge for two to three weeks while stirring or shaking the contents of the jar anytime the thought occurs to you, which should be at least once every day. When stirring, a large wooden spoon may be used effectively.

The cheesecloth should be used to remove the plant matter after the herbs have been allowed to infuse for the appropriate amount of time. The oil should be collected in a glass pitcher. The end of the cheesecloth should be twisted to extract as much oil as feasible from the leafy debris. The next step is to melt pure beeswax (either in a double- boiler on the burner or a Pyrex cup inside a bowl of the glass in the microwaves), and then add it to the infusing oil in an amount of around five parts oils to one component melted wax. This will complete the process. After giving it a stir using a wooden spoon, keep it in a disinfected container made of glass or metal. It is simple to alter the texture of a salve by including a little bit more water to render it more easily spreadable or a little bit more honey to make it thicker or more resistant to spreading. When stored at room temperature away from direct heat and sunshine, a homemade salve that does not include any preservatives will remain used for about six to eight months. When stored in the refrigerator, they have a shelf life of one year or more. The comfrey and plantain salve has a wide range of applications. It will apply to irritated areas such as hives and bee stings, chapped palms and lips, heels with cracks and ragged cuticles, as well as nicks, reductions, and scrapes. It is also wonderful for treating heat rash and diaper rash. One caution after the area has been cleaned and disinfected; you should wait for it to cease bleeding before adding any kind of salve. You should avoid closing in a pathogen of infectious nature.

BOOK 3: Teas and Infusions Made from Medicinal Herbs

Herbal teas are beverages made from medicinal herbs that are steeped in Water and sold as a beverage. They are classified as hydrolysis, which are plant extracts that have been dried using Water, and they are included in the group of plant extracts. Before the turn of the last century, the most common way to consume plants with the purpose of achieving a therapeutic effect was via the consumption of herbal teas.

The term "tisane" refers to a combination of dried and shredded plants (in the form of chopped herbal tea), which are combined in accordance with the concept of synergy among the benefits of each individual herb.

Botanical tea is not technically "tea" despite its name since these drinks often do not include the greens or leaf buds associated with true tea. Herbal tea isn't technically "tea" despite its name since these drinks often do not include the greens or leaf buds associated with true tea. Many of the drinks that are promoted as "herbal tea" and have "herbal tea advantages" are really nothing more than syrupy juice. Is drinking herbal tea healthy for you? Some herbal teas have been used for generations as natural treatments due to the health benefits they give and the fact that they are made from herbs. Herbal teas should be used in moderation and only with the advice of a physician, according to dietitians, since herbal teas might cause some health concerns to worsen in certain people. Steer clear of herbal teas that have sugar or other ingredients added to them. It is not recommended to drink herbal tea in place of seeking professional medical attention.

Herbal teas are completely free of calories and sugar, and they are available in a wide range of mouthwatering tastes. There are many herbal teas that provide health benefits, and recent scientific research has started to substantiate some of the traditional applications of herbal teas.

3.1 Guidelines for an herbal tea's fundamental ingredients

Although herbal tea is often thought of as a straightforward hot beverage to enjoy, it is really a truly medicinal product that occurs when the active compounds found in dried plants are drawn out using Water. Additionally, herbs are paired not only based on flavor but rather according to a highly specific pattern.

•   1-2 plants that enhance and intensify the action of the basic medicine via a synergistic effect or that facilitate the metabolism of the active substances. Additives (Adjuvans 20%).

•   The major impact of herbal tea is caused by 1 to 3 plants, which together make up the basic

Treatment (Remedium Cardinale 60%).

• 1 plant is added as a Supplement (Constituent 10%) to the combination to make it more aesthetically pleasing, particularly in terms of color. The Raspberry and Rosehip berries are two instances of how these berries give the tea made from herbs a lovely shade of vivid red.

• 1 plant called Corrector (Corrigens 10%) enhances the herbal tea's taste and aroma. The principal taste modifiers are anise, fennel seeds, mint, and licorice.

Synergistic effects: Never connect two plants with opposing effects because of the impacts' synergy and antagonistic interactions.

Homogeneity: Always compare the hardness and delicateness of homogenous plant parts (e.g., roots with tree bark, leaflets with flowers; never mix the two since they need distinct cooking techniques).

3.2 Ten Beneficial Herbal Teas That You Ought to Definitely Attempt

Teas made from herbs, such as peppermint oil, Chamomile, and ginger, have a number of beneficial characteristics that might assist in enhancing a variety of aspects of health, including digestion, cardiovascular wellness, and the quantity and quality of sleep.

1. Peppermint tea

2. Chamomile tea

3. Ginger tea

4. Echinacea tea

5. Hibiscus tea

6. Rooibos tea

7. Lemon balm tea

8. Sage tea

9. Rose hip tea

10. Clove Herbal tea

11. Passionflower tea

12. Cinnamon tea

13.   Fennel Tea

14.   Raspberry leaf tea

15.   Nettle tea

3.3 Peppermint tea

Preparation time: 2 Minutes

Making time: 9 minutes

Servings: 1 person

Ingredients

- 8 ounces (250 ml) water

- 7-10 peppermint leaves

- Honey, milk or lemon to taste (optional)

Instructions

Pick between seven and ten peppermint leaves off the root of the plant for every cup of tea that you want to make. When picking leaves, it's best to look for ones that are green as well as spotless. If you purchased a bunch of cut-in-advance peppermints stems, select the leaves that seem to be in the best of health to remove the stems. Do a thorough job of rinsing the peppermint leaves under the running Water. Even if you plucked the peppermint directly from your own yard, you should still thoroughly rinse the leaves to remove any traces of dirt or other contaminants before using them. Smash the peppermint by pressing the leaves between your fingers, which may be done with either your hands or a mortar and pestle.

Peppermint's taste and perfume may be more easily extracted from the plant if it is first broken apart. Smash the peppermint by pressing the leaves on your fingers, which may be done with either your hands or a mortar and pestle. Peppermint's taste and perfume may be more easily extracted from the plant if it is first broken apart. Bring the water to a boil using either an electrical kettle, a kettle that can be placed on top of the burner, or a saucepan. After waiting for the boiling water to reach a rolling boil, turn off the flame and remove the saucepan or pot from where it was being heated. Bring the water to a boil using either an electrical kettle, a kettle that can be placed on top of the burner, or a saucepan. After waiting for the boiling water to reach a rolling boil, turn to stop the heat and remove the saucepan or pot from where it was being heated. After allowing the water to cool for a few minutes and then gently pouring it over the peppermint leaves, the mixture will be ready to use. First, check to see that every leaf is completely covered in the Water, and then cover the cup. Steep the tea for seven minutes if you want it on the milder side.

You should keep the peppermint in the tea for the whole 12 minutes if you want your tea to have a rich peppermint taste and a strong body. After the steeping time for the tea has passed, the tea leaves should be removed. You may either remove them by fishing them out with a wooden spoon or by filtering the brewed beverage into a different cup in such a way that all of the leaves are captured in the strainer. Both of these methods will result in the leaves being removed. Your tea should now be ready to drink. If you like adding extras to your tea, such as honey, milk, or lemon, wait until after you have strained the tea to add them. In any case, I hope you're enjoying that piping-hot cup of mint tea!

3.4 Chamomile tea

Preparation time: 3 Minutes

Making time: 7 minutes

Servings: 2 persons

Ingredients

- 3 tablespoons of Chamomile that have been dried

- 2 cups Water

- Honey, to taste (optional)

Instructions

To get started on the Chamomile tea Recipe, grab a pot and set it over high heat to begin warming up the Water. When the Water reaches a boil, remove it from the heat and stir in the Chamomile that has been dried. Maintain the cover for the next minute. The chamomile tea should now be strained and placed in the tea glasses. Honey should be added to taste (it should just be used as a sweetener; you may totally omit it), and then the dish should be stirred before being served. During the evenings, serve the Chamomile tea recipe with an appetizer.

3.5 Ginger tea

Preparation time: 7 minutes

Making time: 10 minutes

Servings: 2 persons

Ingredients

- A 2-inch piece yields 2 Tbsp.

- 2 ½ Tbsp. chopped fresh ginger

- 2 ½ cups Water

Instructions

In a small saucepan, combine the Water, the sliced ginger, and all of the other ingredients that are optional. Place over high heat and bring to a boil. Once the Water has reached a boil, cover the pot, turn the heat down to medium, and continue to boil the mixture for seven to twelve minutes. After removing the pot from the heat, the taste is going to develop even more. Pour the liquid into cups after passing it through a strainer with a fine mesh. You have the option of sweetening it to taste with the sweetener of your choice and serving it with chopped lemons or oranges. Tea that has been consumed but not put away may be kept in the fridge for up to one week, or it can be chilled and placed in a tray with ice cubes to be used later in beverages such as cocktails, Water with lemonade, tea with ice, or Water. Take note that the ginger taste will become more pronounced as the tea steeps. The ginger, spices, and new Water may be used to make another batch of tea, but it won't have the same level of intensity as the first one.

3.6 Echinacea tea

Preparation time: 3 minutes

Making time: 15 minutes

Servings: 3 persons

Ingredients

- 1/4 cup Echinacea, dried

- 1 tsp mint, dried

- 1 tsp lemongrass, dried

Instructions

First, combine all three of the plants, and then pour 8 ounces of hot water over the mixture. Give the ingredients some time to meld together for around 15 minutes. You may eat this dish simply or with honey.

3.7 Hibiscus tea

Preparation time: 5 minutes

Making time: 8 minutes

Servings: 1 person

Ingredients

- Hibiscus

- Hibiscus pineapple

- Sweetener

- Water

- Herbs

- Whole spices

- Citrus

- Florals

Instructions

Put the petals from the hibiscus flower and the Water that has been chilled in a medium-sized saucepan, then bring the mixture up to a boil around medium-high heat. After the Water has reached a boil, turn the heat down to a simmer and set a timer for ten minutes for the petals to soak. Mix it up every so often. After passing the liquid through a strainer or a colander, the beverage may then be transferred to a big pitcher. Put it in the refrigerator to chill for a while. Then, if you'd like it sweetened, add the sweetener of your choice when it's still hot (add to taste), but only if you wish it sweetened.

3.8 Rooibos tea

Preparation time: 7 minutes

Making time: 10 minutes

Servings: 3 persons

Ingredients

- cups water

- 14 rooibos tea

- 3 cups brown sugar

- 3 tsp honey

- tsp lemon juice

Instructions

In a saucepan of medium size, bring Water to a temperature of medium heat. Once the supply of Water has reached a boil, remove it from the heat. The rooibos tea should now be poured into a teapot. After the Water has boiled, pour it over the tea. It is best to let it sit for around five to six minutes to ensure that the taste of the rooibos tea is completely integrated into the hot Water. After the tea has been made, pour it into individual glasses. Put sugar cubes in it to make it sweeter. To enhance the taste, add a few tablespoons of lime juice and some honey. Tea should be served hot, and you should enjoy it!

3.9 Lemon balm tea

Preparation time: 1 minute

Making time: 8 minutes

Servings: 3 persons

Ingredients

- 1/3 cup of fresh lemon balm leaves

- 1 cup of Water

- 2 tbsps. dried leaves

- 1 tsp lemon juice

- 2 tsp honey

Instructions

Bring one cup of water to a boil in a teapot. Put the zest of the lemon balm herbs in a tea infuser, add the boiling water, and let them steep for at least a minute or longer if you want a stronger cup of tea. Add some honey for sweetness, and finish it off with a dash of fresh juice from a lemon. Enjoy!

3.10 Sage tea

Preparation time: 15 minutes

Making time: 30 minutes

Servings: 3 persons

Ingredients

- 1/2 of an ounce of fresh sage leaves, which is around 45 leaves.

- cups water

- 2 tablespoons sugar

- 3 tablespoons lemon juice

- 1 1/2 teaspoons lemon zest

Instructions

Collect the necessary components. Start the Water boiling in a pot. A low simmer should be maintained for the Water while you add the sage branches, sugar, zest of lemon, and the juice of the lemon. Stir thoroughly. Allow infusing for twenty to thirty minutes or until the desired flavor is achieved, stirring periodically. After that, drain the liquid to remove the sage herbs and the lemon zest. You may serve this dish hot or cold with ice.

3.11 Rose Hip tea

Preparation time: 6 minutes

Making time: 30 minutes

Servings: 4 persons

Ingredients

- 6 cups of Water

- ½ cup (A handful of) rosehip

- 1 tablespoon honey

Instructions

A kettle or saucepan with a cover should have Water poured into it. Toss the rosehips in there as well. Put the cap back on it. Bring everything up to a boil, then reduce the heat to moderately low and let it simmer for 15–20 minutes or until it reaches the desired color and flavor. It should be served in glasses that have been sweetened using a little honey. Pour everything into a jug, add honey, and put it in the freezer to chill until it reaches the desired temperature if you want to drink it cold.

3.12 Clove Herbal tea

Preparation time: 6 minutes

Making time: 30 minutes

Servings: 4 persons

Ingredients

- 1 cup of Water

- 1-4 whole cloves

Instructions

Put one cup of boiling Water and the cloves in a pan and bring to a boil. Bring to a rolling boil. After three to five minutes, turn off the heat source. Strain. If you want your tea to have a sweet taste, you may sweeten it by adding honey to the pot of tea; however, this step is optional. Consuming some of this tea first thing in the morning is the ideal way to experience its full flavor.

Because drinking more than one cup of anything might be harmful to your health, you should make sure that you don't consume more than one cup of this tea. Before including clove tea in your diet, if you are currently receiving any kind of medical treatment, it is imperative that you first discuss this decision with your attending physician.

3.13 Passionflower tea

Preparation time: 6

Making time: 25 minutes

Servings: 2 persons

Ingredients

- 1 cup water

- 1-2 tsp dried passionflower

- 1 teaspoon of an extra herb chosen from the list shown above (this step is optional; if you want to use valerian root, go to the comments section for more instructions).

Instructions

Put one to two tablespoons' worth of the dry herb in the cup. After pouring eight ounces of hot water into the cup with the herb, seal the container with a tiny plate or the top of the cup, and let the infusion soak for twenty to thirty minutes. After the herbs have been removed, strain the liquid and consume it as many as four times a day.

3.14 Cinnamon tea

Preparation time: 4 minutes

Making time: 10 minutes

Servings: 3 persons

Ingredients

- 8 ounces water

- 1 Ceylon cinnamon stick

- 1 tea bag

Instructions

Put the cinnamon stick into the cup, and stir it around. Bring the water to a boil, then pour it into the cup. Infuse the cinnamon branch in the boiling water for ten minutes while keeping the pot covered. Put in the used tea bag. Continue infusing for a further minute or two. Take out the used tea bag as well as the cinnamon stick. Served either warm or very hot.

3.15 Fennel Tea

Preparation time: 4 minutes

Making time: 15 minutes

Servings: 2 persons

Ingredients

- One tablespoon of fennel seeds that have been crushed

- 1/2 teaspoon honey

- 1 1/2 cup water

- 3 mint leaves

- 1/4 inch crushed lightly ginger

Instructions

Bring the Water up to a rolling boil. Put one and a half cups of Water into the saucepan. Allow it to reach a full boil. Next, stir in some ginger and fennel seeds that have been crushed. Allow the Water to simmer over medium heat until the volume has been reduced to one cup. Next, extinguish the gas heat and pour the contents of the pot through a strainer into a cup. Add honey and blend thoroughly. The fennel tea that you ordered is now ready to be served. Your cup of fennel tea is ready and can be served at this time. You may serve it with leaves of mint as a garnish. Have fun with the drink while it's still warm.

3.16 Raspberry leaf tea

Preparation time: 26 minutes

Making time: 6 minutes

Servings: 3 persons

Ingredients

- 6-8 oz. Red Raspberry Leaf Tea

- 1 tbsp. Cashew Butter

- 2-3 Dates

Instructions

To begin, prepare the tea in a vessel as if you were going to make a standard cup of tea. After the tea has finished steeping, transfer it to a blender along with the dates and cashew butter, and process it until it is silky smooth and creamy. Test it out to see whether the sweetness or the amount of creaminess has to be adjusted. Enjoy while it's still warm!

3.17 Nettle tea

Preparation time: 5 minutes

Making time: 13 minutes

Servings: 2 persons

Ingredients

- 1 tablespoon fresh nettle leaves

- Sweetener (brown sugar, agave, or honey) Optional

- 1 teaspoon dried nettle leaves

- 10 ounces of Water

Instructions

A teapot or a tiny saucepan should be used to bring the liquid to a rolling boil. Take the pot off the heat and, using a strainer for your tea, put in the tea with nettle leaves. The leaves should be steeped in boiling water for five to ten minutes. When you steep anything for a longer period of time, the taste will become more concentrated. After removing the tea leaves from the pot, transfer the tea to your chosen vessel. Add sugar if required, and appreciate it!

BOOK 4: Herbal Antibiotics that are Natural

Many lives that would have been lost to bacterial illnesses have been saved by antibiotics. They are created synthetically or from microbes to prevent the development of other germs. They are created by some microbe species, and when they are present in small amounts, they prevent the development of other microorganism species. An alternative definition of an antibiotic is a chemical substance obtained from or generated by living organisms, as well as their synthetic substitutes, which, even in very tiny doses, may impede the life processes of microbes. Antibiotics are very important. However, it is now recommended for any minor issue. That is causing many human bodies to malfunction and digest food improperly. Ironically, it has also weakened people's natural immunity, which will eventually give rise to all kinds of illnesses. With the aid of the most potent natural medicines, illnesses may be treated without causing any damage.

Ever since penicillin became available in 1940, antibiotics have saved countless lives. However, antibiotics were already present in nature at that time. A small number of natural antibacterials have been shown to be quite helpful and efficient in a variety of circumstances. If you decide to utilize these natural antibacterials, speak with your doctor first and describe the signs and symptoms of your illnesses. Because bacterial infections sometimes cannot be treated with natural remedies, and as a result, they spread more and are more difficult to treat. Natural antibiotics have a relatively low risk of adverse effects since they are made from organic materials. Even certain foods have antibacterial effects, and other plants are used to extract essential oils. An extract of cranberries, for instance, has both antibiotic and antioxidant substances. It functions as a natural treatment for infections of the urinary tract (UTIs).

Antibiotics are very important. However, it is now recommended for any minor issue. That is causing many human bodies to malfunction and digest food improperly. Ironically, it has also weakened people's natural immunity, which will eventually give rise to all kinds of illnesses. Ever since penicillin was discovered in 1940, antibiotics have saved countless lives. However, antibiotics were already present in nature at that time. A small number of natural antibacterials have been shown to be quite beneficial and effective in a variety of circumstances. If you decide to utilize these natural antibacterials, speak with your doctor first and describe the signs and symptoms of your illnesses. Because bacterial infections sometimes cannot be treated with natural remedies, and as a result, they spread more and are more difficult to treat. Natural antibiotics have a relatively low risk of adverse effects since they are made from organic materials. Even certain foods have antibacterial effects, and other plants are used to extract essential oils.

Many lives that would have been lost to bacterial illnesses have been saved by antibiotics. They are created synthetically or from microbes to prevent the development of other germs. They are created by some microbe species, and when they are present in small amounts, they prevent the development of other microorganism species. An alternative definition of an antibiotic is a chemical substance obtained from or generated by living organisms, as well as their synthetic substitutes, which, even in very tiny doses, may impede the life processes of microbes. The top organic antibiotics that many all-natural health professionals still employ today are those that our ancestors formerly utilized.

4.1 Raw apple cider vinegar

ACV may aid with weight control, decreasing cholesterol, and reducing the risk of cancer because of its antibacterial and antiseptic characteristics. If you require a topically clean or sterilized wound, you may also use ACV as a free chemical astringent.

Among the advantages of vinegar made from apple cider are:

- Diabetes type 2 prevention.

- Shedding pounds.

- Heartburn relief.

- Minimizing varicose veins.

- Bringing down cholesterol.

- Bleaching teeth.

- Reducing acne.

- Eliminating dandruff.

Recipe

Preparation time: 45 Minutes

Making time: 15 Minutes

Servings: 3 Persons

Ingredients

- 6 to 7 teaspoons of sugar or honey. A single tablespoon is used for each cup of water.

- 6 cups chopped segments, ideally from a variety

- 6 to 7 glasses of warm, but not hot, clean water

Instructions

Mason jars should be 3/4 full of apples or apple leftovers. Warm water with sugar or honey is stirred in. To dissolve, mix. Over the apples, a stream sweetened the water. Leave the highest point of the jar with two to three inches of space. Cover with an elastic band or the screw-top lid from a mason jar, a thin piece of fabric, or a coffee filter. For two weeks, put in a warm, dark location. (Place there and wrap with an absorbent tea towel. This method has a beautiful scent.) After two weeks, sift the particles out while gently pressing on them to obtain more liquid. (At this stage, taste the vinegar. It is really tasty! In essence, it is fermented apple cider. You are going to be able to begin fermenting in a more compact jar when the sediments have been taken out. Wrap in new cheesecloth. For around 4 weeks, put the fermenting vinegar in a warm, dark location. When the apple vinegar made from apples has a distinct apple cider vinegar flavor and aroma, it is finished. If not, let it ferment longer.

Nutrition Facts

Carbohydrates:4g, Fat:1g, Protein:1g, Calories: 14

4.2 Oil of oregano/oregano:

Many people use oregano without recognizing how healthy it is—it's something you can add to the dishes you love in Italian cuisine! It contains antimicrobial characteristics and may aid with weight reduction, yeast infections, and chronic digestive ailments. Caracole, another name for oregano oil, inhibits microorganisms that may cause unpleasant illnesses.

Advantages of Oregano Oil

- It might aid with pain relief.

- It may reduce cholesterol.

- Minimizes inflammation

- Strong antioxidant.

- It could enhance intestinal health.

- It may aid in the treatment of yeast infections.

- Has potential anti-inflammatory effects.

Recipe

Preparation time: 5 Minutes

Making time: 20 Minutes

Servings: 1 Small jar

Ingredients

- 1 cup oregano leaves (dried)

- Jar with lid

- 1 cup olive oil

Instructions

Water in a saucepan is boiling. Turn off the heat when it reaches boiling. Then add the oil that is the carrier and the oregano leaves that have been crushed to the container. After adding the jar to the boiling water, wait 5–10 minutes. After being removed from the water, put the jar in a sunny location for one to two weeks. A few times each week, shake the jar. After the allotted time has passed, filter the leaves oil. Re-insert into the jar. Keep the container of oil in a room that's cold and dark.

Nutrition Facts

Carbohydrates:4g, Fat:1g, Protein:1g, Calories: 14

4.3 Grapefruit seeds crushed with grapefruit seed extract

The dietary supplement citrus seed extraction (GSE) is made from grapefruit seeds, pith, and pulp. To put it another way, some extracts utilize only the seeds, while others use both the fruit and the seeds, and others even include the peel.

Advantages Of Grapefruit Seed

- Mouthwash (to promote healthy gums and teeth)

- Vegetable and fruit wash

- Gargle your throat (to treat colds and aching throats)

- Nasal/sinus wash (for colds and sinus infections)

- Gastrointestinal issues (such as candidiasis and traveler's diarrhea)

- Dropped ears

- Skin injuries

Recipe

Preparation time: 30 Minutes

Making time: 10 Minutes

Servings: 3 Persons

Ingredients

- Cheesecloth or a strainer with fine mesh

- 2 cups of a solvent, preferably at least 80-proof vodka or brandy or vegetable glycerin

- 1 cup of organically grown fresh grapefruit seeds. Gather grapefruit seeds from washed citrus that has been sliced.

- A glass container with a secure cover, ideally made of plastic

Instructions

If you own a Vitamix flour blender, pound the grapefruit seeds in the grinder or blender until they are thoroughly ground (they may be coarse or fine). Alternatively, you may do it the old-fashioned way using a pestle and mortars. Place the ground seeds in a glass jar or plastic container. Ensure that those seeds are thoroughly submerged in the alcohol before adding them to the jar. While some of the crushed seeds may float, daily shaking of the infusion should keep them sufficiently submerged for preservation and infusion. For a minimum of four weeks, put the jar in a cold, dark area after tightly sealing it. A few times each week, shake the jar. After four to six weeks, filter the mixture to get rid of any particles using cheesecloth or a fine-mesh strainer. You may need to strain it twice. It is better to strain food using a wire-connect colander before using a tea strainer with a finer mesh. The extract should be kept in a dark, cool location in a glass container. The extract should remain usable for a number of months. Alternatively, It is better to use transparent containers so that You can monitor the extract's level of freshness. To keep it fresh, it is kept in a cabinet that is dark.

Nutrition Facts

Carbohydrates:4g, Fat:2g, Protein:10g, Calories: 19

4.4 The Honey Spot Healing with Turmeric

Natural anti-inflammatory in nature, anti-septic turmeric is also very efficient in repairing injuries and wounds, decreasing redness, and clearing up acne lesions. Use this DIY spot treatment on the afflicted areas as frequently as necessary or once a day.

Advantages of Turmeric Honey paste

- Boosting the immune system's defenses

- Beneficial for your skin and digestive system

- Essential for losing weight.

Recipe

Preparation time: 10 Minutes

Making time: 5 Minutes

Servings: 3 Persons

Ingredients

- Honey

- jar

- Turmeric

Instructions

Make a paste by combining 1 teaspoon of turmeric powder and a few drops of local organic honey in a small dish. Directly apply the paste to the acne or blemish-affected areas.

Nutrition Facts

Carbohydrates:4g, Fat:0g, Protein:9g, Calories: 7

4.5 Cold-Pressed Coconut Oil

Coconut oil provides a surprisingly wide range of health advantages, including the ability to reduce stress and strengthen the immune system. Capric, lauric, and caprylic acids are abundant in them. It is antifungal, antioxidant, and antibacterial effects come from these omega-3 fatty acids. It may be used to moisturize skin, prepare meals, and cure illnesses. With each of these advantages, it's difficult to see why you wouldn't include coconut oil in your daily routine.

Advantages of Cold-Pressed Coconut Oil

- Natural Energy Booster

- Aids in Weight Management

- Manages Diabetes

- Fights Neurogenerative Diseases

How to make Cold Pressed Coconut Oil

Preparation time: 22 Minutes

Making time: 10 Minutes

Servings: 5 Persons

Ingredients

- About one and a half cups of oil may be extracted from eight coconuts.

- 8 mature coconuts

Instructions

When making coconut cream, you have the option of utilizing either a blender or a juicer as your method of preparation. The approach that uses a juicer will be both quicker and more effective, despite the fact that the food processor's technique is more convenient for most people. After the coconut cream has been prepared, pour it into the container that you have chosen. It is now time to "ferment" the cream so that the curd can be separated from the oil and superfluous water can be eliminated. You may store the cream made from coconuts in a dish or jar for one to two days if you cover it, place it in an area that is warm, and keep an eye on it. There is also the option of wrapping it in a large towel or an extra blanket. We are seeking an atmosphere that is just slightly warmer than normal since this will aid in the fermentation of the coconut, which is necessary to allow for the essential oil to be extracted from the meat of the coconut. After some time has passed, the curds and the oil will begin to separate. The vegetable oil is going to reside on the very top, and the curds made from the coconut will be at the very center. You are going to have some murky water at the bottom inside the container, which you can either throw away or use in stews. It is important to keep in consideration that the fluid will have a taste that is reminiscent of fermentation. Even though this task involves some patience on your part, you should have no trouble scooping out the oil. Take care to scoop out just the oil and leave the curd alone in the container. You may transfer the oil straight into an airtight container that has been cleaned and sterilized. You also have the option of passing the oil via a strainer or a bag designed for nut milk. It is possible to put the curds straight into the filter, and the resulting oil will then trickle into the container you have provided. Remember that there will still be some oil on the filter once you're done.

Nutrition Facts

Carbohydrates:8g, Fat:10g, Protein:19g, Calories: 17

4.6 Ginger Turmeric Tea

Two blooming plant species that are often utilized in herbal remedies are ginger and mustard. Zingiber officinale, more often known as ginger, has a Southeast Asian origin and has been used for many years as a natural treatment for a variety of illnesses. Gingerol, a molecule known to have strong anti-inflammatory and antioxidant qualities, is one of the phenolic chemicals that give it its therapeutic benefits. The identical clan of plants includes turmeric, referred to as Curcuma longa, which is frequently employed as a flavor in Indian cuisine. It includes curcumin, a substance that has been demonstrated to help cure and prevent a number of chronic illnesses.

Advantages of Ginger Turmeric Tea

- Reduce nausea

- Alleviate pain

- Lessen inflammatory

- Support the immune system

Recipe

Preparation time: 10 Minutes

Making time: 05 Minutes

Servings: 3 Persons

Ingredients

- Striped and sliced thinly ginger root, about 1 to 2 inches

- Cut and peeled 3-inch turmeric root

- Water in 6 glasses

- 1 lemon, ideally organic, Meyer

Instructions

The lemon peel should be separated into thin pieces. Lemon juiced, put aside. Mix ginger, turmeric, and the peel of the lemon in a medium pot. Heat the water in addition before bringing it to a boil. Reduce the heat, then simmer for five minutes. Add the juice of one lemon after taking it off the fire and letting it cool a little. If you'd like, mix it with a cinnamon piece!

Nutrition Facts

Carbohydrates:18g, Fat:03g, Protein:12g, Calories: 10

4.7 Honey Made from Fermented Garlic

Making this fermented nectar garlic is the ideal way to strengthen your immune system. You should keep this tasty natural treatment on hand throughout the flu and cold season since honey and garlic each have significant medical advantages.

Advantages of Fermented Garlic Honey

- Reduce the symptoms of asthma

- Assist in treating heart problems

- Boost your immunity

- Used to treat respiratory issues

Recipe

Preparation time: 20 Minutes

Making time: 10 Minutes

Servings: 4 Persons

Ingredients

- 1 cup of unprocessed honey or more as required to completely coat the garlic

- 1 cup of whole, peeled, and gently smashed garlic cloves

Instructions

Put the sliced garlic cloves in a pint-sized Baker's jar with a wide opening. Garlic cloves should be fully covered with honey. Ensure that honey is used to coat them. Put a loose cover on the jar and hide it away in a dim area. Tighten the jar's lid each day or so, then turn it upside down in order to spread the honey over the garlic cloves. When you put it back upright, loosen the cover once more. On the honey appear, you should begin to see little bubbles forming after just a few days to a week. Although you may consume the honey garlic at any time, it will ferment for approximately a month. Over time, the taste will keep evolving, the garlic will smooth out, and the syrup made with honey will become runnier. Keep in a cool location for many months, if not a full year.

Nutrition Facts

Carbohydrates:10g, Fat:20g, Protein:29g, Calories: 27

BOOK 5: Essential Oils Apothecary

Among the different carrier oils, almonds, sunflower, and olive oil are some of the most widely used. These herbs based on oils infusions may be used in balms, soaps, butter, and creams to treat skin conditions. They may also be utilized to condition hair, yet One thing to keep in mind is that herbs that are dried work best for oil infusion. This is when fresh herbs may transfer germs into your oil, causing it to rot, develop mold, or deteriorate since they contain a certain level of moisture. Essential oils are potent, organic aromatic fluids that have a variety of uses, in the use of aromatherapy, personal grooming, spirituality, and other aspects of health and mindfulness.

Contrary to how the term "oil" is used, essential oils don't really have an oily texture. The majority of essential oils are transparent, but others, like orange, lemongrass, patchouli and its blue tansy, maybe amber, yellow, green, or even deep blue in color. By steam or water distillation, fragrant botanicals, including rosemary, lavender, cedarwood, spiked, and cypress, may create essential oils from their leaves, wood, petals, blossoms, needles, bark, or roots. Citrus oil-based products are either cold-pressed or steam-distilled from the peels (peels) of citrus fruits, unlike other essential oils, which are water- or hydro-distilled. Because essential oils are so potent, a little comes a long way. Despite the fact that most essential oils have great scents and are natural, it is crucial to understand and observe essential oil hygiene.

5.1 Advantages of Essential Oils

Essential oils' unique chemical makeup and scent may have beneficial therapeutic effects on both the mind and body. Chemicals that occur naturally make up essential oils. Linalyl ester and Linalol are components of entirely natural lavender oil for aromatherapy, for instance. When the term "chemical" is used in relation to essential oils, some people who are unfamiliar with dealing with them may feel perplexed and afraid. There are no additions of any type in pure essential oils. Nevertheless, pure essential oils do include naturally occurring compounds, commonly known as components. Essential oils that are administered topically undiluted or improperly diluted might cause skin sensitivity or irritation. Some may also be phototoxic when improperly diluted. Essential oils must be mixed with a carrier oil, such as jojoba, honey almond, or apricot kernel oil, before topical use. For further in-depth details on carrier oils, see the section under "Carrier Oil Profile."

Since the molecules of the essential oil enter the respiratory tract and get absorbed into circulation, careful breathing may also have medicinal benefits. Diffusers, inhalers, and scented jewelry are a few ways to inhale. The majority of the time, extremely few bottles of essential oils are marketed for individual usage. Both the price and the quality of essential oils may vary substantially. The uncommonness of the particular botanical, the nation of source and growing/climate circumstances, the distiller's quality requirements, and the quantity of oil the botanical produces are all variables that may impact the quality as well as the cost of the oil. Numerous essential oils may be found in mixtures that can be bought. You may save money by buying pre-made essential oil blends rather than having to purchase each essential oil separately. You may benefit from utilizing mixes created by skilled aromatherapists and craftspeople when you buy blends from seasoned, reliable essential oil providers. Essential oils might be useful for:

- Boost work performance by lowering stress and improving focus.

- Boost your mood.

- Boost your sleep.

- Lessen your pain and worry.

- Annihilate viruses, fungi, and bacteria.

- Cut the inflammation.

- Headache relief.

- Decrease nausea.

5.2 Some Vital Oils and their Benefits:

There are multiple essential oils are available; each and every oil has its own benefit and uses. Some of the basic oils are listed and explained below:

1)   Tea Tree Essential Oil

Tea tree oil is an amazing essential oil that has a wide variety of remedial and curative capabilities. It is additionally referred to as melaleuca fluid, which is considered to be one of the best natural oils for treating a variety of skin and hair conditions. Melaleuca oil has been used for centuries. This essential oil, which is endowed with potent antibacterial, antiviral, anti-inflammatory, antifungal, and nourishing properties, is effective in the prevention of bacterial and fungal disorders that affect the skin, hair, and nails. Tea tree oil has a variety of other applications, including those of natural mouthwash, insect repellant, and deodorant. Tea tree oil, when applied topically to the skin, may cure and treat typical skin disorders, in addition to improving the skin's general health.

The Advantages and Applications of Tea Tree Essential Oil

- Repellents for insects

- Hand disinfectant

- Organic antiperspirant

- promote healing of wounds

- To treat small cuts and scratches, use an antiseptic

- Clear up zits

- All-purpose cleaner mouthwash that doesn't include chemicals

- Fungus on the nails, be gone!

- Soothe irritation of the skin

- Athlete's foot treatment

- Suppress hair flakes

- Eliminate mold from produce.

- Antiviral

- Treat Psoriasis

Preparing Tea Tree Oil

Depending on where you are located, this may be somewhat challenging. In the USDA's plant hardiness zones eight through eleven, you may cultivate and buy Melaleuca alternifolia. The little tree might be found in other tropical places via gardening shops or periodicals. The greatest stills are made of glass or stainless steel, although these materials may be pricey.

Make sure that you have a level surface that is close to an electrical outlet yet situated in a secure location that children and dogs cannot access. An extinguisher for fire and a wastebasket should always be kept handy. Essential oils are potent substances that should not be handled or inhaled

Directly under any circumstances. The higher the component concentration, the more powerful the end product. Throughout the whole procedure, it must be between thirty and seventy-five percent filled at all times. Re-establish the connection between it and the distillation unit. When you are shopping for a distillation set on the internet, you might find online marketplaces that sell boiling stones made of a material other than Teflon. When the water is boiling, this prevents it from breaking through the condensation set and destroying the process. In order to determine the ideal quantity of leaves to utilize for your distillation apparatus, you may find it necessary to carry out some trials and errors.

Because of this, the oil will be able to flow inside the conduit. In order to begin the process of steam distillation, you will need to turn on the hot plate. Please be patient as the plate heats up and the water works its way through the leaves. They will begin to contract as they are stored in the container. Within the first half an hour, the bulk of the oil has to be extracted and transferred to the container located at the opposite end of the process. When you are through distilling, make sure the hot plate is turned off. The water should be separated from the oil in the vessel that was used to collect the essential oil. Put the oil of the tea tree into a dropper bottle with a dark-colored tint. In order to acquire additional essential oil, you will need to replace the plant material and continue the procedure.

2)   Lavender oil

To make lavender oil, first, soak dried flowers of lavender in an oil carrier of your choice for at least a week and up to a few weeks. This process yields the most potent oil. The natural aromatic compounds of lavender are taken out of the dried flowers and into the oil that serves as the carrier as the lavender is allowed to infuse in the oil. Virgin olive oil, jojoba oil, oil from sweet almonds, and many other types of oils are examples of popular possibilities for carrier oils. A moment from now, we are going to quickly go over the distinctive qualities and advantages of around a dozen various carrier oils in order to assist you in narrowing down the sort of oil that you will utilize.

Pure lavender oils, which are produced by a distillation extraction procedure as opposed to infusion, are not the same as this kind of DIY lavender oil. Although there are several small stills for the home and hobbies, distilling is most often carried out on an extensive industrial scale. In addition, just a little quantity of oil is produced from a tremendous amount of lavender blossom material. The technique we're employing in this lesson, however, may produce a sizable volume of oil from lavender with many fewer blossoms!

The Advantages and Applications of Lavender Oil

One thing is common knowledge: lavender has a pleasant aroma. That's how fantastic it is. The oils and salve are my go-to's for a natural "cologne," and I adore diffusing organic essential oils of lavender to uplift the atmosphere of our house. Lavender's calming fragrance has long been used to treat mental health issues, including stress, sadness, and sleeplessness. Still, it's capable of so much more!

Lavender oil is a popular component in many homemade insect repellents because of its reputation for warding off unwanted visitors like insects and flies. Lavender's medicinal properties extend well beyond its aromatic application, both topically and orally. Lavender has been shown in scientific research to have pain-relieving, anti-inflammatory, antibacterial, antifungal, and antioxidant properties. It also aids in the healing of wounds and the restoration of damaged skin. As a result, it works well to treat a wide variety of skin conditions, including eczema, stings, scars, acne, bites, burns, and acne scars. You may now comprehend the popularity of lavender's inclusion in all sorts of organic skin care products.

- Allergies
- Acne
- Anxiety
- Athlete's Foot
- Asthma
- Bruises
- Chicken Pox
- Burns
- Colic
- Cystitis
- Cuts
- Depression
- Dysmenorrhea
- Dermatitis

- Earache

- Headache

- Flatulence

- Hypertension

- Insect Repellent

- Insect Bites

- Itching

- Migraine

- Labor Pains

- Oily Skin

- Scabies

- Rheumatism

- Scars

- Sprains

- Sores

- Strains

- Whooping Cough

- Stretch Marks

- Stress

- Vertigo

Lavender Oil Preparation Methods

The oil infusion technique may be used to manufacture homemade lavender oil quite easily. All you have to do is gently pack dried or pure lavender flowers into a glass jar, filling it from halfway to the top. You may use individual lavender flower heads or the full head. Furthermore, the majority of publications advise using dried lavender flowers or buds, but I love using fresh ones!

If you take one easy step, you won't have any mold problems, and you will be able to observe the distinction in the oil that produce as a result. If you utilize dried blossoms, you might want to think about using a pestle and mortar to slightly crush the lavender. The lavender bits' surface area will expand, giving them more surface area to interact with the oil. After that, add your preferred carrier oil on top of the dried flowers in a clean container. Oil should be poured into the glass until it reaches the jar's lip within a half-inch. You want to decrease the air in the container while still leaving space for the contents to shake since oxygen and oil don't make good friends. Use a lid to close the jar.

3)   Oil of Peppermint

The peppermint plant, which grows in North America as well as Europe between water and spearmint, is the source of peppermint oil. In addition to being used as a scent in soaps and beauty products, peppermint oil is often utilized as a flavor in meals and drinks. Additionally, peppermint oil is utilized locally as a moisturizer or ointment and consumed orally as a dietary supplement for a number of medical ailments. According to clinical data, peppermint oil may be able to relieve irritable bowel syndrome indications. Additionally, it could alleviate indigestion and stop GI spasms brought on by either endoscopy. According to certain studies, using it topically may help relieve tension headaches and breastfeeding-related cracked nipples. However, additional study is required to substantiate these findings. Dietary supplements and topical treatments, including peppermint oil, are probably safe for the majority of people when taken as recommended.

The Advantages and Applications Oil of Peppermint

Traditional herbalists may employ peppermint for the following purposes:

- Halt itchiness

- Destroy germs

- Lessen pain

- Assist in the body's mucus elimination and minimize muscular spasms

- Decrease or avoid vomiting

- Decrease bloating

- Increase blood flow

- Encourage sweating

Peppermint Oil Preparation Methods

Only the wide, green leaves should be used. A peppermint plant may die if its stems are removed. Peppermint oil, in contrast to other kinds of essential oils, is really an infusion. This implies that how much you finally have will depend on how much oil as a carrier you apply to soak your leaves. Pour a steady flow of water over the fallen leaves in a pitcher or mesh strainer to wash away the dust, dirt, and debris. You may also let your peppermint soak for five to ten minutes in a small basin for additional thorough cleaning. Lay the leaves out in one layer on a tabletop, chopping board, or another flat surface after giving them a little shake to get rid of any extra water. To prevent the leaves from bending or twisting as they dry, you may smooth them with the palm of your finger, if required. The leaves may be crushed with a mallet, mortar and pestle, or even using the tip of a spoon against a firm, hard surface. You should use mild, uniform pressure when moving your utensil. The leaves should be collected and put on the bottom of the container.

As numerous leaves as you can fit into the container, but be careful to allow space at the top for the materials to be moved around a little. Only enough oil should be used to thoroughly cover the peppermint. When finished, shake the jar to move the leaves about and aid in better integrating them into the container of oil. Place the jar in a corner of your cooking area, bathroom, pantry, or veranda after tightly sealing it. As long as the place isn't too hot or cold, it will function everywhere. It's also beneficial to maintain the fluid out of sunlight directly for this reason.

Get rid of the jar's lid once the peppermint has steeped for the night, and cover the opening with cheesecloth. To allow the oil to escape through the cheesecloth, lay the jar over a different container. After that, hand-pick up as many scattered leaf fragments as you can. The same method you used for the first set of leaves should be used for the second bunch, with only sufficient force to shatter the outermost layer and release the oils within. Prevent chopping or shredding the leaves into impractically tiny bits. On as many occasions as necessary, repeat the preceding procedures to make your oil the required strength. This normally takes a few days, but you may keep adding fresh leaves for as long as a week. Once closed, the jar will aid in keeping your oil fresh until you're ready to apply it. Keep your oil at or just below ambient temperature in a dark, cool place to extend its shelf life. Also, remember to quickly reseal the jar after each use.

5.3 Other Types of Oils

On a scale that ranges from 1 to 5, oils are ranked according to their comedogenicity. Those ingredients that fall closer to the bottom of the pyramid are known as "non-comedogenic" and are the ones that are least likely to cause your pores to get clogged. 3 indicates a high likelihood, and 5 indicates an extremely probable possibility that your pores may get clogged. The skin may be revitalized, nourished, and hydrated with the aid of the crucial omega fatty acids that are found in all of these oils in large quantities. You might also build your own unique mixture by combining a few different oils in the appropriate proportions.

1)   **Almond Oil Sweet:** On the comedogenicity scale, sweet almond oil ranks at a two, making it an excellent option for dry and delicate skin, especially the skin of babies. Jojoba and grape seed oils rank at one, making them somewhat more effective moisturizers. It is effective in treating excessive sebum production, inflammation, scarring, eczema, and dryness on the skin. Additionally, the use of sweet almond oil helps lessen the appearance of dark circles under the eyes and helps maintain an even complexion. It may be eaten; however, it is recommended that you do not heat it.

2)   **Vinegar Oil:** Acne-reducing properties of grape seed oil include its antibacterial properties and extremely low comedogenic rating (1). It absorbs well and is neither oily nor heavy. It is a decent option for oily skin, even if it might not offer as much hydration as some of the other lubricants on the list. It may be consumed cold or at ambient temperature; however, high-heat cooking is not advised.

3)   **Oil of Jojoba:** Despite having a rating of 2, jojoba oil is still regarded as non-comedogenic. Because it has a chemical structure with the natural oils on our skin, it is thin, non-greasy, and absorbs quickly. Jojoba oil is a fantastic choice for oily or mixed skin since it helps to break apart and eliminate excess sebum! Jojoba oil is so effective at clearing clogged pores and eliminating pollutants that some individuals first suffer a "purge" (small outbreaks). Additionally, studies demonstrate that it reduces inflammation and aids in wound healing. It's very extended shelf life of as many as five years is a bonus. Jojoba oil should not be consumed.

4)   **Virgin Extra Olive Oil:** Virgin extra olive oil is a little thicker than other of the drier oils on the list and is much more moisturizing and nutritious for dry skin. It is a fantastic option for multipurpose lavender oil since it is edible. It is a two on the comedogenic scale; however, if used excessively, it might sometimes lead to breakouts in those with acne-prone skin. An anti-aging substance known as hydroxytyrosol, a unique antioxidant found in EVOO, protects the skin from

free radical damage.

5)   Rosehip Seed Oil: Important vitamin E, fatty acids, and vitamin A are abundant in rosehip seed oil and help to speed up cell turnover. Scars may be healed, and fine lines and discoloration can be reduced. Rosehip Seed oil is light and readily absorbed, scoring a two on the comedogenic meter. It has a shelf life of just six months and is not advised for internal usage.

6)   Avocado Oil: Despite its thick, greasy consistency, avocado oil is an excellent deep moisturizer. While avo oil is known for its ability to soften the skin, it may also help reduce scars, irritation, and age spots. It's non-toxic and comes in at a comedogenic level of 3.

7) Hemp Seed Oil: When compared to the other carrier oils we've looked at, Hemp Seed Oil has the lowest comedogenicity score: a whopping 0! It has similar amino acids and fatty acid composition to our natural skin oils; therefore, it is easily absorbed by the skin despite being a very light, "dry" oil. In addition to being a fantastic topical option for all skin types, hemp oil may also be consumed.

8)   Coconut Oil: The natural beauty community sings the praises of coconut oil. It has potent antibacterial, antiviral, antifungal, and anti-inflammatory activities because of the presence of caprylic acid and other chemicals. Although it has many uses, virgin coconut oil may be difficult to work with for infusions due to its solid state at ambient temperature and rather high comedogenic rating (four). Fractionated coconut oil, on the other hand, is a liquid at ambient temperature (making it ideal for infusions) and is far less prone to cause pores to get clogged.

9) Argan Oil: Argan oil, commonly known as Moroccan oil, is very mild and hydrating, and it also has a comedogenic score of zero. You may find this oil in a wide variety of cosmetics, although it is most often used in hair care products. Argan oil has beneficial effects on the skin, including protection from UV rays, reduction of fine wrinkles and excessive oil production, skin softening, and maybe the treatment of stretch marks. Argan oil comes in both ingestible and non-ingestible varieties. Currently, my favorite facial oil is argan oil.

10)   Sunflower Seed Oil: Similar to Safflower, also oil, Sunflower Seeds Oil has many of the aforementioned benefits. Vitamin E is a strong antioxidant that helps protect skin from sun damage and heal damaged skin. There are medium, high, and low varieties of oleic acid in sunflower seed oil. Selecting a low-comedogenicity oil can almost eliminate the possibility of breakouts. Sunflower oil may be consumed.

11)   **Safflower Oil:** Both oily and acne-prone skin types, as well as dry, irritated skin, may benefit greatly from the use of safflower oil. It has a comedogenic rating of 0 and a low weight, yet it has a significant amount of moisturizing and healing properties. The use of safflower oil may help unclog pores and maintain a healthy balance of natural oils in the skin. However, those who are allergic to members of the ragweed species should stay away from this oil. It may be consumed at temperatures that are low as well as high without losing its edibility.

BOOK 6: The Plants

6.1 Gum Arabic / Babhul

The venerable old acacia plant has been honored for a considerable amount of time. One of the most beneficial byproducts of the acacia plant is gum Arabic, which in Asia is known by the name babul. Gum Arabic has a long history of use in Ayurveda medicine as well as many other types of traditional medicine. When it was initially utilized as a binding agent in the culinary industry, gum Arabic was prized for its curative effects. However, its applications have since expanded well beyond that. Since that time, Gum Arabic has seen widespread application in the production of some of the most sugary condiments and foods that humanity is familiar with. When we get into the medical advantages of gum Arabic, let's first find out what all the commotion is about. An excellent source of dietary fiber may be found in the gum that is produced by the Acacia Dakar tree. It is also known as Senegal gum, Indian gum, acacia gum, and gum Sudani. Acacia gum is another name for it. This plant is rather prevalent in the western and coastal regions of India. There are a variety of uses for it thanks to its high level of solubility in water.

The Health Advantages of Gum Arabic

- Guard Yourself Against the Dangers of Diabetes

- Excellent for Maintaining and Improving Heart Health

- Analgesic for aching muscles and joints

- Helps with weight reduction efforts.

- Beneficial for your gut health

- Best for the control of your gut

- Syndrome intestine irritable due to diabetes

- Managing high cholesterol levels

6.2 Corn cockle

Corn cockle is really a unique kind of herb. Both the root and the seed are used in the medicinal process. Corn cockle is used even though there are severe questions over its safety for the treatment of fluid retention, cough, menstruation problems, worms, and jaundice (yellowing of the skin). Corn cockle seeds are occasionally administered straight to the skin in order to cure malignancies, warts, tumors, and inflammation of the uterus. Additionally, corn cockle seeds are used in order to cause swelling of the cornea and conjunctiva of the eye. Both hemorrhoids and exanthemata, which are rapid skin breakouts produced by an infectious viral or bacterial infection, may be treated by applying the root topically to the affected area.

The Health Benefits of Corn Cockle

- Tumors.

- Cancers.

- Warts.

- Resulting in an increase in the size of the eye's conjunctiva and cornea.

- Uterine enlargement caused by pregnancy.

- Breakouts on the skin.

- Fluid retention.

- Hemorrhoids.

- Cough.

- Worms.

- Menstrual problems.

- Jaundice.

6.3 The Acacia Tree

Acacia is a kind of plant that can be found in large quantities in North America and is known to have a wide range of positive effects on one's health. Acacia is a kind of plant that has blooms that are a brilliant yellow hue with a top. It is used to treat a wide variety of conditions, including congestion, colds, diarrhea, fever, illnesses of the gall bladder, smallpox, and TB, among others. Acacia is also known as the "Thorn tree" and "Wattle," among other common names. There are many different species of Acacia; however, the most common one includes leaves that are a dark green color, branches that are thorny, and flowers that are yellow. The shittah tree, the wood which was utilized in the construction of the Tabernacle, is most accurately identified as the common acacia tree. Because of the foliage and fruit, you can tell that acacia is receiving water despite the fact that you virtually never see any water surrounding the tree itself. This is a fascinating occurrence that occurs with acacias. Because of the tree, you may deduce that there is water at that location. If God is the source of living water while we constitute the plant that receives it, then others around us will be able to tell by the fruit that we produce whether or not we are receiving living water. How well we fare in the desert is directly proportional to the amount of water that we have access to.

The Health Advantages of the Acacia Tree

- Helpful in Treating and Preventing Sore Throats and Reducing Cholesterol

- Acacia Provides Advantages to Oral Health

- Diabetes Treatment Skin Disease Treatment Diabetes Treatment

- Acacia as an Aid in the Treatment of Digestive Issues

- Acacia may help with weight loss in a number of ways.

- Acacia acts as a detoxifier and cleanser for the body while simultaneously boosting the immune system.

6.4 Camel thorn

Because of the positive effects, it has on one's health, camel thorn, also known as Alhagi pseudalhagi and more popularly as Yavasa or Javasa, is considered to be of considerable therapeutic value in Ayurveda. This plant grows to a considerable height, and its root system is rather extensive. The Central Asian region is home to a significant population of this perennial plant. In the nation of India, it is cultivated to a large extent in the Ganges valley, the mountains of India, and Kashmir, in addition to some regions of Jaisalmer and Gujarat. It is often said that consuming this plant will result in significant gains in one's physical prowess.

The Health Benefits of Camel Thorn

- Camel thorn for the treatment of respiratory conditions

- Beneficial effects of camel thorn on sexual health

- Camel thorn for the purpose of achieving healthy weight gain

- To aid with digestion, camel thorn

- Arthritis treatment using camel thorn

6.5 Rose of Jericho

It is an old plant that has been around for a long time and is famous for its capacity to "come back to life" when it seems to have dried up and passed away. People in many regions of the world, including the Middle East, different sections of Europe, and even farther afield, utilize it as a traditional medicine to treat a broad variety of illnesses. These include aches and pains associated with menstruation, labor and delivery, arthritis, and metabolism and respiratory conditions like diabetes and asthma, among others. People also put it in holy water and utilize it for psychological and religious rituals to protect themselves from disease and bad energy. In other cases, the holy water is just plain water. The primary flower is an upright blooming plant that may reach a height of up to 30 centimeters (12 inches) in height. It is interesting to note that some also perceive it as a tumbleweed owing to the fact that it resists drying out so incredibly well. In point of fact, it can make it through even the driest of environments. The rose of Jericho will dry out and coil up into a ball like a tumbleweed if it is placed in an environment that is comparable to a desert and has very little rainfall. It hibernates in this state so that the blooms it contains on the inside are preserved. This behavior continues until it is provided with water.

The Health Benefits of Rose of Jericho

- Reduce the level of blood pressure.

- Improve both your general health and the quality of your sleep.

- It was said that it was highly beneficial in the treatment of pregnant women.

- Tea may be made from the plant's dried leaves, blossoms, and seeds, or its oil can be processed into holy water. The herb can also be used to produce holy water.

- The herb was utilized as a treatment for common ailments like asthma, the common cold, and the stiffness associated with arthritis.

6.6 Leek

However, although most chefs are familiar with onions and garlic, a significant number of them have never worked with leeks. Leeks are members of the allium family, much like their more well-known relatives, onions. Leeks have the appearance of enormous green onions and may be used in many of the same ways as onions.

The Health Benefits of Leek

- Full of plant chemicals that are to our benefit.

- Include a wide range of nutritional components.

- It may have anti-inflammatory and cardioprotective effects

- It may reduce the risk of developing certain malignancies

- It may be helpful for weight reduction

- It may be beneficial to the digestive system.

- Vitamin K is found in abundance in leeks.

- Solid Structures

6.7 Horseradish

Horseradish is a type of root vegetable tree that is well-known for both its strong flavor and pungent aroma. It has a long history of usage around the globe, dating back thousands of years, most often as a seasoning but also for medical uses. This root includes a number of chemicals that have been shown to have potential health advantages, such as antibacterial and anticancer activities. It is generally agreed that horseradish was first cultivated in Eastern Europe. It belongs to the same family as mustard greens, wasabi, broccoli, cabbage, and kale; it is a cruciferous vegetable. It is distinguished by its long, white root as well as its green foliage. After the root is sliced, an enzyme begins the process of converting a substance known as sinigrin into mustard seed oil. It also has the potential to irritate the nose, eyes, and throat. In order to prepare the root to be utilized as a condiment, it is normally grated and then preserved in a mixture of vinegar, salt, and sugar. This kind of horseradish is called prepared horseradish. There is also a version of horseradish sauce that incorporates mayo or sour cream into the recipe.

The Health Benefits of Horseradish

- Enhances the immune system.

- Possible cancer-fighting properties

- Contains elements that inhibit bacterial growth

- Natural ability to boost the health of the respiratory system

- The metabolism may be sped up by using a weight loss aid.

- Antibacterial treatment improves circulation and eliminates mucus buildup.

- Facilitates the digestive process.

6.8 Agarwood

Numerous health advantages and the treatment of a wide range of illnesses have been attributed to the usage of agarwood in its numerous incarnations, including oil, wood, powder, and the plant itself. Ayurvedic, Tibetan, and other traditional forms of East Asian medicine are among those that continue to make use of agarwood as a therapeutic ingredient, even though the practice dates back thousands of years.

The Health Benefits of Agarwood

- Pain, including that caused by rheumatic and arthritic conditions, may be relieved with agarwood oud oil.

- Achieve Calmness Within Yourself With Agarwood and Oud Oil

- Additionally, agarwood oud oil can help the digestive system.

- Agarwood and oud are beneficial to the skin.

- Get Rid of Your Halitosis With Agarwood and Oud Oil

- Agarwood and oud for the treatment of breast cancer

- Agarwood oud can also be used to spice up your love life.

- Agarwood oud may be used to enhance meditation; it can also help regulate menstruation and alleviate symptoms of premenstrual syndrome (PMS). Agarwood and oud might help relieve itching.

- To Help Alleviate the Pain of Gout, Agarwood and Oud Oil

- Coughs may be alleviated with the use of agarwood oud oil, which also helps with congestion.

6.9 Some Other Plants and Their Uses

Plant Name	Uses
Orchid	aid in the prevention of cancer, boost the body's defenses and enhance vision.
Angelica	used to treat intestinal gas (flatulence) and heartburn
Basil	assist in reducing anxiety and sadness
Bergamot	utilized for joint discomfort, mental clarity, and anxiety
Chamomile	Used for gastrointestinal issues, hay fever, inflammation, muscular spasms, menstruation issues, sleeplessness, ulcers, and wounds

Pot marigold	Used to treat a wide range of illnesses, such as fever, jaundice, stomach ulcers, conjunctivitis, and liver issues. Wounds and burns
Borage	used for coughs and fevers
Anise	use anise for migraines, constipation, and indigestion
Bay leaf	Treating renal congestion, inflammation, and blood dysentery
Caraway	as a carminative, appetizer, galactagogue, and treatment for pneumonia and indigestion
Chervil	skin freshener, diuretic, expectorant, and digestive aid
Mugwort	digestion issues, menstrual irregularities, or elevated cholesterol levels
Coriander	used to treat constipation, bacterial or fungal infections, and anxiety
Mugwort	used to treat hypertension, period irregularity, severe stomach issues
Dandelion	The roots of dandelion may be used in order to cleanse both the liver & bladder.
Meadow clary	applied to brush teeth as well as treat throat inflammation.
Dill	treating stomach ailments, colic, hiccups, bad breath, flatulence, and hemorrhoids.
Chives	utilized for treating gastrointestinal problems, soothing sore throats, and growing hair
Meadowsweets	recommended to treat heartburn, which is ulcers, digestive issues, pneumonia, and influenza
Marjoram	Problems of the alimentary tract, the eyes, the nose, the heart, the rheumatoid system, as well as the nervous system.
Thyme	usage to get rid of coughing, congestion, and gas in the stomach

Mint	Might Enhance Cognitive Functioning
Rosemary	epilepsy, hysteria, rheumatic pain, stomachache, spasms, nervous agitation, dysmenorrhea, improved recall
Nasturtium	Nasturtium leaves are a potent antibacterial and may be applied to wounds to assist with fighting infection.
German Chamomile	lowers swelling, quickens the healing of wounds, eases muscular spasms, and acts as a kind of sedative to aid with sleep.
Oregano	Utilized as an anti-bacterial, anti-inflammatory, menstrual problem treatment, diabetic, gastrointestinal (diarrhea, indigestion, stomachache), and respiratory (asthma, bronchitis, cough) medication.
Lemon Balm	Improve appetite, promote sleep, lessen stress and anxiety, and soothe stomach pain and discomfort (including colic, gas, and bloating).
The Great Yellow Gentian	utilized to treat digestive issues such as heartburn, bloating, diarrhea, and lack of appetite. Additionally, it is used to treat fever and stop muscular spasms.
Globe Artichoke	decrease gas, cramps, and nausea. Additionally shown to decrease cholesterol and safeguard the liver these substances.
Echinacea	Infections of the urinary tract, vaginal yeast (Candida) sickness, otitis media (also known as athlete's foot), sinusitis, and hay fever (also known as allergic rhinitis), and even slow-healing wounds may all be treated with echinacea.
Ashwagandha	boosts memory and increases how well the brain and neurological system work. It promotes a healthy sexual & reproductive balance by enhancing the reproductive system's functionality.

Great Burdock	diabetes, gout, acne, extremely dehydrated skin, psoriasis, fluid retention, fever, anorexia, and stomach disorders.
Lemon Grass	treating gastrointestinal spasms, indigestion, heartburn, hypertension, convulsions, pain, nausea, coughing, aching joints (rheumatism), a high temperature, a common cold, and fatigue. Additionally used as a mild antibiotic and to destroy bacteria.
Rosemary Sage	enhance cognition, immune system function, and muscular pain
Sagargota, Bonduc nut	Helps to lessen the symptoms of a fever, such as stomach pain, joint inflammation, and organ edema or swelling.
Elder	Elder leaves and berries cannot be used to cure respiratory problems, including pneumonia, colds, coughs, & fever. However, elder blooms may.
Costus	used to treat a wide range of medical conditions, particularly those characterized by inflammation, including chronic gastritis, stomach ulcers, rheumatoid arthritis, asthma, & bronchitis.
Thyme	Thyme's chemical composition may help in the treatment of bacterial and fungal infections. Additionally, due to its antioxidant characteristics, it could lessen coughing. There is widespread use of thyme to treat coughs, dementia, and loss of hair in patches caused by alopecia areata, but there is not any conclusive scientific evidence to support it.
Khus	Improves Heart Function, Treats Disorders of Sleep, Treats Inflammation, Treats Pain, Improves the Nervous System, and Boosts Immunity. Eczema is a skin disorder that is treated. It may be utilized in a number of culinary contexts.

Rui leaves	Rui leaves may be made to ignite a sore region by dabbing castor oil, melted butter, or other oils on them. B. Place one drop of the rui juice from its leaves into the ear to treat an earache.
Vitex Negundo	anticancer, antibacterial, antimicrobial, antifungal, and anti-inflammatory effects.
Yarrow	Utilized in cancer, toxicity caused by chemotherapy, healing wounds, skin inflammation, spinal cord injury, bowel dysfunction, infections caused by bacteria, respiratory viruses including COVID-19, anxiety, regulating blood sugar levels in type 2 diabetes, protecting the liver & gallbladder, and wound healing.
Sorrel	beneficial for swells and diseases associated with inflammation. Treating injuries such as boils, sores, chickenpox, and bruises.
Stevia	utilized to increase the heartbeat, treat retention of water, decrease blood pressure, and treat diabetes, heartburn, and excessive blood uric acid levels.
Tarragon	used to treat symptoms including indigestion (dyspepsia), low appetite, postoperative vomiting and nausea, sleep issues, toothaches, and various other ailments.
Marsh Mallow	Used to soothe the stomach & throat by coating them. Additionally, it is utilized therapeutically to relieve chapped skin.
Chamomile	used to treat a variety of human conditions, including hay fever, inflammation, muscular spasms, irregular menstruation, sleeplessness, ulcers, as well as wounds, digestive issues, pain from rheumatic arthritis, and constipation.

Celery	effectiveness for aches and pains in the joints and muscles, Gout, anxiety, and headache, stimulation of the appetite, Exhaustion, retention of fluid control of bowel motions, use as a sedative for sleep, Gas, enhancing digestion, reducing breast milk production, and other disorders.
Siberian Ginseng	utilized to boost energy, vitality, and lifespan, as well as prevent colds and the flu.
Parsley	Use parsley to treat a variety of ailments, including urinary tract infections (UTIs), kidney calculi (nephrolithiasis), digestive system (GI) issues, constipation, and skin diseases.
Sea Buckthorn	help wounds heal more quickly, control blood sugar, fight cancer, and be useful for skin care
Elder	used to treat conditions of the lungs, including bronchitis, coughs, colds, and fever. Tea made from elderflowers encourages perspiration, which may decrease fever.
Gum Arabic Tree	Excellent for enhancing heart health. Take Measures to Avoid Diabetes. Relief for joint and muscle pain. Favorable to your bowels Lose weight, and it's best for your stomach.
The Acacia Tree	Acacia is used to treat a variety of health issues, including digestive issues and dental problems, help people lose weight, relieve sore throats, lowering cholesterol, improve the body's defenses, treat type 2 diabetes, and treat skin conditions.
Camel thorn	Use camel thorns to heal respiratory diseases and sexual health. Camel thorn for arthritis, and healthy weight growth, For digestion, use camel thorn.
Leek	Use to lower inflammation and strengthen the heart, Use to support good digestion, prevent some malignancies, and assist with weight loss; beneficial for healthy bones, Leeks contain a lot of vitamin K.

Rose of Jericho	Use to maintain lower blood pressure and improve general health and sleep quality. It was said to be quite beneficial for prenatal care. Asthma, the common cold, and agony from arthritis were all treated with the herb. The plant is generally processed to create holy water from its oil or tea from its drained leaves, petals, and seeds.
Agarwood	Banish Bad Breath Using Agarwood Oud Oil, Support Your Digestive System With Agarwood; Also Oud Oil to enhance skin health, and Breast Cancer Treatment With Agarwood Oil Add Agarwood Oud to Your Love Life to Spice It Up. To improve meditation, control menstruation, and ease itching, use agarwood oud. Agarwood oud can assist with a cough, relieve congestion, and reduce gout pain.
Horseradish	offers possible anti-cancer advantages, is used to improve respiratory health, and has antibacterial properties. Increases blood flow, has a built-in antimicrobial defense, and aids in clearing mucus. Use as a supplement to boost metabolism, promote immunity, help with digestion, and lose weight.
Corn cockle	In the treatment of cancer. Fill in the Tumors. Reduce Warts to Uterine Swelling. Causing the cornea and conjunctiva of the eye to enlarge. Hemorrhoids, fluid retention, and acne. Good for worms, irregular menstruation, jaundice, and cough.
Cactus	Addressing obesity, diabetes, excessive cholesterol, and hangovers.
Eucalyptus	utilized to clear congestion on the tip of the nose and chest. Help relieve throat discomfort, as well as cure bronchitis and sinusitis.

BOOK 7: Common Disorders and Pathologies

Any aberrant state of one's body or brain that causes pain, malfunction, or anguish not just to the individual afflicted but also to all who come into touch with the individual in question. Injuries, impairments, syndromes, symptoms, aberrant behaviors, and atypical differences in structure and function are often included in the scope of the word when it is used in its broadest sense. A deviation from the typical or typical functioning of the brain or body. Genes, diseases, or traumatic experiences may all have a role in the development of disorders. Disorders of mental health, which are often referred to as diseases, have an effect on the thoughts, feelings, and actions of persons who are affected by them. Even if there is no clear connection between genetics and the likelihood of developing a mental disease, a person's way of life, which includes their diet and the amount of physical activity they receive on a regular basis, may play a part in the development of mental health concerns such as depression and anxiety in that individual. Disorders of mental health may either be short-term or long-term conditions. And they impact an individual's capacity to interact with other people and to carry out day-to-day activities. Even while there are certain things that may be done to enhance general mental health, there are other problems that are more significant and could need the help of a professional.

7.1 The most Prevalent forms of Mental Illness

- Mood Disorders

- Anxiety Disorders

- Conditions Classified as Psychotic

- Eating disorders

- Dementia

7.2 Mood Disorders

A mental health problem known as a disorder of mood is one that predominantly impacts an individual's emotional state. It's a condition where you go through extended stretches of either excessive happiness or intense depression, or both of those emotions. Anger and impatience are two of the other persistent feelings that might be associated with certain mood disorders. It's natural for your disposition to shift based on what's going on around you. However, in order to get a diagnosis of a mood illness, symptoms must have been present for at least a few weeks.

Why do people have mood disorders?

Researchers think that a number of variables, including the following, contribute to the appearance of mood disorders:

Genetic factors: Individuals who are carriers of a strong family record of a mood illness are more inclined to acquire mood disorders themselves, which demonstrates that mood illnesses are likely to be partially genetic/inherited in nature.

Biological factors: The amygdala and the cortex of the orbitofrontal are the regions of the brain that are responsible for regulating your moods and emotions. Imaging studies of the brain have shown that those who suffer from mood problems have a larger-than-normal amygdala.

Environmental factors: Stressful life transitions, such as the loss of a loved one; persistent stress; traumatic occurrences; and abusive treatment received as a kid are significant risk factors for the emergence of a mood illness later on in life, particularly depression. There is a correlation between depression and chronic diseases such as Parkinson's disease, type 2 diabetes, and heart disease.

What signs and symptoms are associated with mood disorders?

Each kind of mood disorder is characterized by its own unique set of symptoms and/or patterns of signs. Mood disorders generally manifest themselves with symptoms that have an impact on a person's state of mind as well as their ability to sleep, eat, maintain their energy level, and think clearly (such as having racing thoughts or an inability to concentrate).

In general, these are some of the signs of depression:

- An absence of energy or a sluggish sensation may be present.

- Experiencing feelings of sadness for most of the period or virtually every day.

- Experiencing feelings of worthlessness or hopelessness.

- Having suicidal or death-related thoughts.

- A diminished desire to participate in activities that earlier offered pleasure.

- Difficulty staying focused on what's going on around you.

- A loss of hunger or an inability to control eating.

- Either getting too much or too little sleep.

7.3 Anxiety Disorders

Anxiety disorders are a subtype of mental health conditions that may affect a person. If you suffer from an anxiety disorder, then you might experience feelings of dread and terror in response to certain items and circumstances. You can also notice physical manifestations of your worry, such as your heart racing and your palms becoming sweaty. It is not abnormal to have some level of nervousness. If you need to solve an issue in the workplace, go to a conversation, take an exam, or execute an important choice, you can have feelings of anxiety or nervousness. And some people really benefit from having anxiousness. For instance, anxiety enables us to recognize potentially harmful circumstances and concentrates our attention, allowing us to avoid harm. However, an anxiety disorder is very different from the occasional feelings of worry and mild panic that some people experience.

Causes of Anxiety Disorders?

Women are more likely to suffer from anxiety problems than males. Researchers are still attempting to figure out why that takes place. It's possible that it's caused by the fluctuating levels of hormones that occur in women, particularly throughout the menstrual cycle. Additionally, the hormone testosterone could play a role; males have more of it, and some research suggests that it helps reduce anxiety. There is also the possibility that women may be less inclined to seek therapy, which results in a worsening of anxiety. The symptoms of anxiety disorders are similar to those of other types of mental disease. They are not the result of human frailty, defects in one's character, or difficulties in one's upbringing. However, experts aren't quite certain about what factors lead to anxiety disorders. They have a hunch that a number of other elements are involved, including the following:

Environmental factors: Anyone who was born with a greater risk for anxiety disorders, to begin with, may be more susceptible to developing the condition after experiencing a traumatic event.

Chemical imbalance: The chemical equilibrium that regulates your mood might be altered when you are under intense or persistent stress. An anxiety disorder may develop as a result of prolonged exposure to high levels of stress over a period of time.

Hereditary factors: Hereditary factors have a role since anxiety disorders often run in families. Eye color is one trait that may be inherited from either one or both of your parents.

- **Symptoms of an Anxiety Disorder**

- When something stirs up your emotions, you often respond in an exaggerated manner.

- When someone's worry gets in the way of their daily life, they may be suffering from an anxiety disorder.

- You can't control your answers to events.

Different types of anxiety disorders are associated with a unique set of symptoms. The following are some examples of general symptoms associated with anxiety disorders:

Mental symptoms

- Nightmares.

- Being overcome with feelings of terror and unease.

- Thoughts that are difficult to regulate and compulsive.

- Recurring thoughts or memories of tragic events that occurred in the past.

Physical symptoms

- A sensation of dry mouth.

- Hands that are either cold or sweaty.

- Feelings of being out of breath.

- Racing or fluttering heartbeats.

- A numbing or tingling sensation in the hands or feet.

- Nausea.

- Muscle tightness.

7.4 Psychotic Disorders

The separation from reality is the hallmark of psychosis. People are prone to having erroneous thoughts as well as experiences that are not genuine. Psychosis is not a disorder in and of itself. It is a word that is used to describe a number of different symptoms.

The following are two main categories of psychosis:

- **Delusions:** These may be incorrect beliefs that an individual clings to with great tenacity, despite the fact that other people do not believe them, or there is a great deal of evidence to suggest that a belief is not correct. Delusions of control may lead a person to think, for instance, that their thoughts or actions are being remotely controlled by another person.

- **Hallucinations:** When this happens, sections of your brain make the mistake of acting as they might if your senses (sight, hearing, smell, touch, and taste) were picking up on everything that was truly occurring. Hearing sounds that are not there is a manifestation of an auditory hallucination, which is one kind of hallucination.

What are somewhat the most typical triggers that lead to psychosis?

Psychosis is a sign that is associated with a wide variety of mental health problems. The following conditions are included in the group referred to as "Schizophrenia Scope and Similar Psychotic Disorders":

- Brief psychotic disorder.

- Schizophrenia.

- Substance/medication-induced psychotic disorder.

- Schizophreniform disorder.

- Delusional disorder.

- Schizotypal (personality) disorder.

- Schizoaffective disorder.

- Psychotic disorder due to another medical condition.

It is also possible to develop psychosis in conjunction with some forms of mood disorders. These are the ones:

- Major depression, manic-depressive illness

- Other illnesses connected to depression

There are a variety of medical problems that may lead to psychosis

Additionally, psychosis may be brought on by a broad variety of different illnesses that have an effect on both the brain and the body. These are the following:

- Hormone-related illnesses such as Addison's disease and Cushing's disease, as well as situations in which the thyroid system is either overactive or underactive.

- Dementias other than Alzheimer's disease, such as vascular dementia.

- Infections of the cerebral cortex or spinal cord, known respectively as encephalitis and meningitis.

- Lyme illness.

- Lupus.

- Multiple sclerosis.

- Stroke, as well as other neurological diseases (those connected to the brain).

- Postpartum psychosis, which is a severe form of postpartum depression that affects a very small percentage of new mothers.

- Deficiencies in vitamin B1, often known as thiamine and vitamin B12.

Other factors that might lead to psychosis

There are a variety of causes that might give rise to psychosis or symptoms that are strikingly similar to those of psychosis. Due to the rapid onset of psychosis, the underlying reasons may more accurately be described as triggers in some instances. In other cases, it could be a drawn-out procedure. The following are examples of situations or causes that may contribute to the development of psychosis:

- Severe injuries to the head, including migraines and traumatic brain damage.

- Stress or anxiety levels that be unexpectedly high.

- Misuse of booze, prescription pharmaceuticals, or recreational substances (the condition described earlier is characterized by behavior that persists over a longer length of time).

- Traumatic events (past or current).

What signs and symptoms are associated with psychosis?

In most cases, it is not simple to recognize the early warning indications of psychosis. It's possible that they'll show up a week before the rest of the symptoms, depending on what caused the psychosis in the first place. These symptoms may take a variety of forms, depending on the underlying reason. The following are some of the most prevalent early warning indicators of schizophrenia, which is a disorder that always includes some type of psychosis:

- Alterations in behavior (difficulty concentrating or thinking, avoiding things that are typically done).

- Shifts in sociability, including a withdrawal from family and friends.

- Alterations in their emotional state, such as appearing fearful, suspicious, or frightened, or a discernible reduction in how often they display their feelings.

7.5 Eating disorders

Eating disorders are significant problems that may have a negative impact on a person's emotional as well as physical health. These disorders include issues with the way that you consider dietary habits, volume, and shape, as well as difficulties with the way that you actually consume. These symptoms have the potential to impact not just your physical health but also your mental state and your capacity to operate in significant facets of life. Eating disorders have the potential to become lifelong struggles and even, in extreme situations, may lead to death if they are not successfully treated. Anorexia, bulimia, and the disorder of binge eating are the three eating disorders that are seen most often.

What are the underlying factors that lead to dementia?

It is unknown what exactly triggers eating problems in people. As is the case with other forms of mental illness, there are a variety of possible reasons, including the following:

Biology: Eating disorders may be caused, at least in part, by biological reasons such as changes in the brain's chemical composition.

Genetics: There is evidence that the genes of some individuals make them more likely to develop eating problems.

Most Frequent Forms of Biological Illnesses

1)   Cystic Fibrosis

Cystic fibrosis, sometimes known as CF, is a genetic disorder that leads to the accumulation of thick, sticky mucus in many organs, including the lungs and the pancreas. In individuals who do not have cystic fibrosis, the mucus that coats the organs and cavities of the body, such as the airways and the nose, is greasy and watery. If you do have cystic fibrosis, the thick mucus that builds up in your airways makes it difficult for you to breathe. Additionally, mucus obstructs the passageways in the pancreas, which leads to difficulties in the digestion of food. It's possible that infants and children with cystic fibrosis won't be able to derive enough nutrients from the food they eat. In addition to affecting your sex organs, liver, sinuses, and intestines, cystic fibrosis is a chronic and progressive disease that lasts a long period and becomes worse over time.

What are the factors that lead to cystic fibrosis (CF)?

There is a hereditary component to cystic fibrosis. Individuals who are affected by cystic fibrosis inherit two defective genes, one from every one of their parents. Because one has to have two different gene variations in order to develop the ailment itself, cystic fibrosis is considered to be a recessive disorder. (An earlier word for gene variation is gene mutation.)

In patients with cystic fibrosis (CF), which signs could they experience?

- Stools that are greasy or loose.

- The inability to thrive is defined as the failure to gain weight while having a healthy appetite and consuming the appropriate number of calories.

- Difficulty in breathing.

- Infections of the lungs often occur (recurrent bouts of pneumonia or bronchitis).

- Frequent episodes of wheezing.

- Recurring infections in the sinuses.

- A sluggish rate of development.

- A persistent cough.

2)   Albinism

Albinism is a very uncommon hereditary condition in which a person is born without a typical quantity of pigment called melanin in their skin. Melanin is a substance that is produced in your body and is responsible for the pigmentation of your eyes, skin, and hair. The majority of individuals who have albinism have extremely pale skin, hair, and eyes. They are more likely to suffer from sunburns and skin cancer as a result. Because melanin plays a role in the formation of optical nerves as well, you can have issues with your eyesight.

What are the reasons for albinism?

Mutations in certain genes are to blame for albinism since these genes are the ones in charge of melanin synthesis.

What signs and symptoms are associated with albinism?

The signs and symptoms that follow may be experienced by those who have albinism:

- Areas of the skin that are without pigment.

- Skin, hair, and eyes that are very pale.

- A condition is known as strabismus (eye crossing).

- Vision issues.

- Rapid eye movement (nystagmus).

- Sensitivity to light is often known as photophobia.

3)   Autoimmune Disorders

The organs and cells that make up the immune system are responsible for defending your body against outside invaders, such as bacteria, parasites, viruses, and cancer cells. An autoimmune illness is caused when the immune system mistakenly attacks the body rather than defending it from harmful substances. It is not known why the immune system behaves in this manner. There are around one hundred different autoimmune disorders currently identified. Lupus, rheumatoid arthritis, Crohn's disease, and ulcerative colitis are some of the more common autoimmune diseases. Autoimmune illnesses have the potential to impact a wide variety of tissues and almost every organ in the body.

What triggers autoimmune illnesses?

It is still uncertain what the specific etiology of autoimmune disorders is. On the other hand, there are some variables that might put you at a greater risk of developing an autoimmune illness. These are some of the risk factors:

- Having family members who have been diagnosed with an autoimmune illness. There are illnesses that are hereditary and tend to run in families.

- Several different drugs. Have a conversation with your healthcare practitioner about the potential adverse effects of the blood pressure drugs, statins, and antibiotics you are taking.

- Smoking.

- Being exposed to harmful chemicals.

- Suffering from at least one autoimmune condition already. Because of this, the likelihood of you contracting another illness is increased.

- Being feminine — Women make up 78% of those who are diagnosed with an autoimmune illness.

- Infections.

- Obesity.

What are the signs and symptoms of an autoimmune disease?

- Soreness, stiffness, and edema in the joints

- Aches and pains in the muscles

- Weakness in the muscles

- Bloating.

- Inflammation

- Constipation.

- Acid reflux.

- Abdominal discomfort.

- Nausea.

- Blood or phlegm in the feces (also known as poop).

- Allergies to certain foods.

4)   Pathology

The study of disease, and more specifically of the structural anomalies that are caused by illness, is called pathology. The origin of the term pathology may be traced back to two Greek words: pathos, which means "suffering," and -logia, which means "the study of." The term "pathology" may refer to both the study of illness as well as the features of the illness itself (for example, "the pathology of cancer"). Pathology may additionally be employed to describe the qualities of the study of illness. Anatomical pathologists, clinical disease, and genetic pathology are the three primary branches that fall under the umbrella term "pathology."

The Beginnings of Pathology

The study of pathology may be traced all the way back to the beginning of time. One of the oldest known societies to chronicle sickness and its impact on parts of the body was the ancient Egyptians. They did this as early as 3000 BC. Papyrus scrolls from antiquity offer information about a variety of ailments, including cancer, fractures of the bone, parasitic organisms, and tumors that might or might not have been cancer. Later on, beginning in the fifth century, before Christ, the Greek surgeon Hippocrates made a significant impact on both the field of medicine and the field of pathology. Hippocrates was the source of inspiration for a large number of ancient Greek writers, and these authors documented extensive knowledge about wounds, tumors, and illnesses such as TB. Additionally, the practice of dissecting animals started at about this time. The concepts of Hippocrates eventually made their way to Rome. Even if scientific advancement as a whole slowed down throughout the Middle Ages, Byzantine and Arab doctors nonetheless made important contributions to the field of illness research.

The invention of the telescope in the nineteenth century was responsible for the most significant advancement in pathology. It was not until recently that cells were able to be examined in exquisite detail. In order to better understand the illness, researchers shifted their attention from examining complete organs to researching individual cells. Pathology research grew at an exponential rate once microscopes were invented and made more widely available. This led to significant advances in the medical and scientific fields, such as the capacity to transplant organs and tissues.

Different kinds of pathology

Anatomical pathologists, clinical pathologists, and genetic pathology are the three primary subspecialties that fall under the umbrella term "pathology." These subgroups may be further subdivided into even more precise divisions; pathology is a varied discipline due to the wide variety of illnesses and approaches to the study of diseases that are out there.

a.   Molecular Pathology

The study of anomalies in cells and tissues at a molecular level is what is known as molecular pathology. It is a wide category that is employed to describe the investigation of illness that may affect any tissue or organ in the body by evaluating the molecules that exist in cells. This research falls under the umbrella term of "molecular pathology." It is possible for it to incorporate components of anatomical pathology as well as clinical pathology. The polymerase chain reaction (PCR), which may be used to multiply DNA, fluorescent labeling, and species imaging of chromosomal and DNA microarrays (small quantities of DNA deposited onto biochips), are some of the methods that may be used in the field of molecular pathology.

b. Clinical Pathology

Through the examination of physiological fluids and tissues in a laboratory setting, clinical pathology is able to identify diseases. For instance, the chemical makeup of a sample of blood may be studied, in addition to the cells and the identification of any microorganisms, such as bacteria, that might exist in the blood. Laboratory science and clinical pathology are two names that are sometimes used interchangeably to refer to the same area of study. The following are examples of important types:

• **Hematology:** like chemical pathology, is concerned with the investigation of blood, but unlike chemical pathologists, the primary focus of hematology is to determine the cause of various blood illnesses. Additional components of the hematopoietic network that are investigated by hematologists include the lymphatic system and the bone marrow.

• **Clinical chemistry:** often known as chemical pathology, is the process of determining the chemical composition of physiological fluids by means of testing and microscopes. The investigation of blood and the immunological components found within it, such as white blood cells, is a typical component of biological pathology.

• **Immunology:** often known as immunopathology, is the investigation of diseases that affect the immune system. It covers topics such as the immune system's reactions to foreign molecules, which are allergies, immunodeficiencies, and the denial of organ transplants.

c. Anatomical Pathology

The investigation of anatomical aspects, such as tissue extracted from the body or even a whole body in the event of an autopsy, in order to diagnose illness and expand understanding of it is known as anatomical pathology. The study of anatomical pathology may include studying cells using a magnifying glass, but it additionally includes examining organs in general (such as a spleen that has burst, for example). In addition to this, research into the chemical characteristics of cells, including the immunological markers they express, is also included. Anatomical pathology may be broken down into a few main subfields, which are as follows:

- **Cytopathology:** Cytopathology is an investigation of tiny groups of cells that are either shed in physiological fluids or collected by scraping. One example of this would be the cells that are retrieved during a Pap smear for the cervical region. Cancer of the cervical cavity and some kinds of infections may both be detected with a Pap smear. The cervix is swabbed in order to collect the cells, which undergo further processing and analysis before being seen via a microscope in order to look for any abnormalities.

- **Examining:** with the use of a microscope, tissues that have been dyed with a dye in order to make them more apparent or observable are what constitute histopathology. Antibodies are often used in the process of labeling distinct cellular components with fluorescent dyes or dyes of varying hues. Following the broad use of the microscope in the field of pathology, a wide variety of techniques were developed for preserving and coloring tissue.

- **Surgical pathology:** The study of tissues that have been taken from a patient after surgery is referred to as "surgical pathology." The inspection of a tiny amount of tumor tissue to identify whether the growth is aggressive (cancerous) or benign, as well as to establish a diagnosis, is a frequent example. A biopsy is the term given to this particular technique.

5) Hemophilia

Hemophilia is an uncommon blood illness that may be passed down through families. It is characterized by a decreased ability of the blood to clot, which can lead to an increased likelihood of bleeding or scarring. Hemophilia is a condition that occurs when your body does not produce sufficient proteins (clotting factors) to assist in the process of your blood clotting. Proteins in the bloodstream are responsible for the clotting process. They collaborate with the platelets in your blood to produce clots that stop bleeding after an injury. The risk of bleeding is increased when clotting factor levels are low. The missing factor is that clots may be replaced as part of the treatment for this illness provided by medical professionals. Although there is no cure for hemophilia, those with the condition who are able to manage their condition with medication often live almost as long as those who do not have the condition. Genetic counseling and replacement therapy for genes are two innovative treatments for hemophilia that are currently being investigated by medical professionals.

What are the signs and symptoms of hemophilia?

The most concerning symptom is abnormal or excessive hemorrhage or bruising. Individuals with bleeding may have substantial bruising even after sustaining relatively small injuries. This is an indication that they are bleeding under the skin. They may bleed for an exceptionally long period of time, either that's bleeding after an operation, bleeding after dental treatment, or just bleeding from a wounded finger. They can begin bleeding for no obvious reason, such as unexpected bloody noses.

Whether a person has severe, mild, or moderate hemophilia determines the severity of their tendency to bruise easily and bleed easily:

Individuals with intermediate hemophilia who have major injuries can vomit for an exceptionally long period. Individuals with serious hemophilia frequently experience unintentional bleeding or gushing for no apparent cause. Individuals with a minor form of hemophilia may have abnormal bleeding, although this complication often manifests itself only after significant surgery or damage.

Other symptoms that might occur include the following:

• Your brain is starting to bleed. Extreme cases of bleeding in the brain, which may be fatal, only very infrequently occur in people who have severe hemophilia. Brain bleeds may result in recurrent headaches, double vision, or a feeling of extreme sleepiness in the patient. Seek immediate medical attention if you have bleeding and are experiencing any of these symptoms.

• Soreness in the joints as a result of internal bleeding. You may have discomfort, swelling, or a warm sensation in the joints of your ankles, ankles, hips, and shoulders.

What are the root causes of hemophilia?

Some genes are responsible for the production of clotting factors. The genes that hold the instructions for creating normal clotting factors may alter or change in individuals who have inherited hemophilia. It is possible that the altered genes may deliver instructions that will result in the production of aberrant clotting factors or an insufficient number of clotting factors. However, around twenty percent of all instances of hemophilia are spontaneous, which means that a person has the condition even when there is no history of excessive bleeding in their family.

7.6 Dementia

The term "dementia" refers not to a particular illness but rather to the condition of a person's mental function at a given time. A loss in cognitive abilities from a previously greater degree that is severe enough to cause problems with day-to-day functioning might be considered dementia. Dementia is characterized by this deterioration. A person has dementia if they have more than one of the particular issues listed above, including a decrease in the following areas:

- Reasoning.

- Memory.

- Language.

- Mood.

- Coordination.

- Behavior.

Infections and disorders may damage some regions of the brain, leading to the development of dementia. These regions are responsible for memory, learning, decision-making, and language. Alzheimer's disease is by far the most prevalent reason why people get dementia.

On the other hand, additional recognized reasons for dementia comprise the following:

- Dementia involving Lewy bodies, often known as DLB.

- Conditions that are similar to dementia but are caused by reversible factors, such as the adverse effects of medicine or thyroid issues.

- Vascular dementia.

- Frontotemporal dementia.

- Alzheimer's disease is the underlying cause of dementia.

- Mixed dementia.

What are the underlying factors that lead to dementia?

Damage to the brain is what leads to dementia in a person. The nerve cells in your brain are what are affected by dementia, which in turn impairs your brain's capacity to communicate effectively with its different regions. The blood supply to your brain may get obstructed, depriving your brain of the oxygen and nutrition it needs, which can also lead to dementia. Brain tissue cannot survive in an environment devoid of oxygen and nutrition. Depending on the region of your brain that was damaged, you may have a variety of symptoms as a consequence of the damage. Certain forms of dementia cannot be treated and often become worse over time. Other forms of dementia are brought on by other medical disorders that have an impact on the brain. An additional cluster of health problems may bring on symptoms that resemble dementia. The symptoms of dementia may be reversed in many cases, and the diseases that cause dementia can be treated.

What are the different signs that dementia is present?

•   Making the same observations or asking the same questions several times in a very short amount of time.

•   Having trouble remembering recent occurrences or information.

•   Losing track of objects that are often used or putting them in unexpected places.

•   Struggling to find the appropriate words to describe what's going on.

•   Being unaware of the current year, month, or season.

•   Going through a shift in one's disposition, conduct, or interests.

The following are some indications that dementia is progressing:

•   You will have an even more difficult time remembering things and making judgments.

•   It gets more challenging to communicate effectively and find the proper words.

•   Activities of daily living that were formerly simple, including brushing one's teeth, getting an espresso of coffee, using a TV remote, preparing food, and paying bills, become increasingly difficult to do.

•   A reduction in your capacity for reasonable thought and action, as well as your ability to find solutions to problems.

•   Alterations in one's normal sleeping routine.

•   An increase in the severity of symptoms such as anxiety, frustration, bewilderment, agitation, suspiciousness, melancholy, and/or depression, as well as a worsening of these symptoms.

•   Requiring a greater amount of assistance with tasks related to everyday living, such as personal hygiene, using the restroom, bathing, and eating.

- Having hallucinations, which include seeing people or things that aren't really there in the environment.

These are some of the most common symptoms associated with dementia. Dementia may affect various parts of a person's brain, which is why people with the same diagnosis might have quite distinct sets of symptoms. Certain varieties of dementia are characterized by a distinct set of symptoms in addition to those of the more common types.

BOOK 8: DIY Remedies and Wellness

There are a number of home remedies that may be used to treat a wide range of conditions, including discomfort, swelling, and colds. Research doesn't always back up these claims, however. However, there is evidence from research suggesting that some could be effective.

8.1 The anti-inflammatory and digestive benefits of mint

Although it may seem like an everyday herb, mint is really rather complex. It is possible for it to give a variety of applications and advantages, depending on the kind. You should seek Wintergreen if you are experiencing pain since it contains methyl salicylate, a chemical that may operate in a manner similar to that of capsaicin. Before it begins to have its numbing operation, applying it may feel like a pleasant "burn" on the skin. This action is helpful for reducing discomfort in the joints and muscles. Peppermint is the other variety of mint that is often used in traditional practices of medicine. Peppermint, which is an element in a wide variety of various treatments, has been shown to be particularly useful in assisting in the treatment of IBS (irritable bowel syndrome) symptoms. In the colon, peppermint stimulates an anti-pain way, which in turn decreases inflammatory discomfort in the digestive system. This is perhaps the reason why it works so well in treating irritable bowel syndrome. A peppermint essential oil capsule or cup of peppermint tea may be beneficial for treating headaches, influenza, and other body aches and pains in addition to digestive and stomach issues.

8.2 Oil of eucalyptus, used for the treatment of pain

There is a substance in eucalyptus oil known as 1,8-cineole that has the potential to alleviate pain. When studied on mice, the substance had effects similar to those of morphine. Proven source. And those of you who are enthusiasts of essential oils, you've been in luck. It has been scientifically shown that inhaling eucalyptus oil may alleviate aches and pains throughout the body. If you're a fan of Vick's VapoRub and have been using it as a home cure for congestion, you should know that eucalyptus oil is the secret component that makes it work. However, not everyone can benefit from breathing in eucalyptus oil the same way. This oil has the potential to aggravate asthma and might be hazardous to pets. Infants may also have difficulty breathing as a result of this condition.

8.3 Shiitake mushrooms to help you out in the long run

A liquid form of shiitake mushrooms contains lentinan, which is referred to as the active compound hex-associated compound (or AHCC for short). At the level of the cell, it fosters antioxidant and anti-inflammatory activities, according to a reliable source. Research in Petri dishes reveals that AHCC may aid with suppressing breast cancer tissues, and its relationship with the body's immune system may assist in fighting cancer by boosting immune systems that have been compromised by chemotherapy. If you find that drinking bone broth helps you relax, try adding some chopped shiitake mushrooms the next time you make it. After a period of four weeks, those who consumed between 5 and 10 grams of shiitake mushrooms on a daily basis saw improvements in their immune systems.

8.4 Aloe vera may be used to provide moisture

The leaves of the tropical plant known as aloe vera each secrete a transparent gel when the plant is harvested. It has been shown that the topical use of aloe vera gel may assist in the fight against germs, reduction of inflammation, and promotion of wound healing. Psoriasis, rashes, wounds, and burns are just some of the skin ailments that benefit from using this remedy because of its anti-inflammatory properties. Lupeol, urea-based nitrogen-containing compounds, cinnamonic acids, and sulfur are all found in aloe vera, and they all work together to prevent acne by inhibiting the growth of germs that may lead to breakouts. The effectiveness of clove-basil oil as a treatment for acne was investigated when varying quantities of gel made from aloe vera were added to the oil. The lotion's effectiveness in reducing the appearance of acne was directly correlated to the amount of aloe vera that it contained. According to the findings of another research, the combination of tretinoin cream and aloe vera gel containing 50% was much more efficient in removing acne than tretinoin cream used on its own. A treatment for acne that is derived from the antioxidant vitamin A is called tretinoin cream. Even while the gel made from aloe vera by itself was not successful in treating acne, when combined with tretinoin cream and clove-basil oil, it significantly improved the condition of the patient's skin. It's possible that using aloe vera gel on its own might help clean up acne, but it could work even better when paired with other treatments or pharmaceuticals.

The best way to apply aloe vera gel to treat acne

1.   Using a spoon, take the gel outside of the aloe vera leaves.

2.   When you put other treatments for acne to your skin, additionally apply the solution to your

face. You may try combining it with the other therapy you are using and then applying the resulting mixture to your skin. Alternatively, you might start with another acne treatment and then apply the aloe gel on top of it.

3.   Perform the procedure once or twice a day or more often as needed.

8.5 Ginger, used for relieving aches and nausea

When you catch a cold or throat infection or are suffering morning sickness and nausea, it is virtually required that you try ginger. The preparation of a cup of tea is rather routine: If you want a more potent impact, grate the ginger into your tea. The usefulness of ginger as an anti-inflammatory agent is another advantage of ginger that receives less attention than the others. Try some ginger next time you get a headache and feel a bit nauseated. Ginger will help. Ginger has an effect that is distinct from that of other pain medications that focus on inflammation. It prevents the production of certain inflammatory components and reduces inflammation already present by using an antioxidant that has a reaction with the acidity that is present in the fluid that is found between the joints. Its anti-inflammatory properties are accompanied by none of the negative side effects that are associated with the use of nonsteroidal anti-inflammatory medications (NSAIDs).

8.6 Topical use of green tea

Green tea has many health advantages, and many people consume it. But it also has positive effects when administered topically. The flavonoids and tannins in green tea have been shown to be effective in combating inflammation and acne-causing bacteria. Epigallocatechin-3-gallate (EGCG), an antioxidant found in abundance in green tea, has been demonstrated to decrease inflammation, sebum production, and P. acnes development in those with acne-prone complexions. When acne sufferers apply a green tea extract with a concentration of 2% to 3% to their skin, their sebum production decreases, and their acne clears up dramatically. There are a few green tea-based skincare items on the market, but it's easy and affordable to whip up your own at home.

8.7 Capsaicin for aches and pains

This active ingredient of the chili pepper has been used for centuries in traditional medicine, and it is just now gaining popularity outside of homeopathy. Capsaicin has recently gained popularity as an effective topical pain reliever. The affected region of the skin will become more heated and then numb as the treatment progresses. Qutenza is a capsaicin patch available with a prescription; it has very high concentrations of the active ingredient. So, if you have some cayenne pepper or hot peppers on hand and you're experiencing persistent muscular pain or body aches in general, use them! Create a cream containing capsaicin. To give your coconut oil a more refined appearance, beat it with a handheld mixer until it turns light and fluffy. Before utilizing the substance extensively, it's best to see how your body reacts to it. You might also use jalapeno peppers; however, their level of spiciness would vary. Wear gloves while applying, and avoid getting the lotion in your eyes or on your face.

8.8 Honey water and lemon juice

When combined with lukewarm water, honey and lemon juice may do miracles for your skin. The antifungal properties of lemon juice were discovered naturally. Additionally, the Vitamin C in it aids in skin renewal and stimulates the production of new, healthy skin cells. In contrast, honey's antibacterial and anti-inflammatory characteristics do more than only eliminate excess oil from the face; they also unclog pores, which may be a contributing factor in acne.

8.9 Baking soda

Baking soda may be used as a fast, inexpensive, and easily accessible treatment for dandruff. Dead skin cells are shed, and itching and scaling are calmed thanks to their purported exfoliating properties. Because of its antifungal qualities, it may also be useful in treating dandruff. Previous research conducted in test tubes indicated that after 7 days, baking soda fully suppressed fungi development in 79% of samples from some of the more frequent strains of fungi that cause skin diseases. In another earlier research, 31 patients with psoriasis were tested for the effectiveness of baking soda. The itching and discomfort caused by the condition were much diminished after just three weeks of treatment with baking soda-based baths. However, further studies are required since baking soda was shown to have no impact on psoriasis, skin moisture, or skin redness in a single study. Apply the paste to damp hair and massage it into the scalp for optimal results. Leave it in for a minute or two, then proceed with your regular shampooing routine.

8.10 Coconut water and Turmeric Milk

Indians have always revered coconut water as a refreshing beverage. Skin wrinkles and wrinkles may be minimized with regular consumption of a glass of pure coconut water first thing in the morning. It's a natural way to keep your skin supple, elastic, and hydrated.

The health and beauty advantages of turmeric milk have been recognized for decades. As an antibacterial and antiviral, it has also found application in traditional and Ayurvedic medicine.

BOOK 9: Plant-based Recipes

9.1 Creamy Veagn Coleslaw

Preparation time: 20 Minutes

Making time: 10 Minutes

Servings: 4 persons

Ingredients

- One tablespoon of Dijon mustard

- Six tablespoons of vegan or without eggs mayonnaise

- A single tablespoon of cider vinegar

- 1 cup of shredded carrots, which is equal to around 2 medium carrots.

- A quarter of a teaspoon of the seeds of caraway or celery seeds.

- 1 teaspoon sugar

- A little bit of salt

- 2 cups of red cabbage that has been finely sliced

- A little bit of ground black pepper

- 2 cups of green cabbage that has been finely sliced

Instructions

Mustard sauce, mayonnaise, vinegar, and sweetener should all be mixed together in a big basin. To taste, season with pepper, salt, and seeds of caraway (or celery seed). Toss the mixture after adding the red cauliflower, green cauliflower, and carrots.

Nutrition Facts

Calories: 115g, Fat:10g, Carbs:6g, Protein:1g

9.2 Black Bean-Quinoa Bowl

Preparation time: 10 Minutes

Making time: 05 Minutes

Servings: 5 Persons

Ingredients

- 2/3 cup of cooked quinoa

- A quarter cup of rinsed canned black beans

- 2 tablespoons of fresh cilantro that has been chopped

- 1/4 cup of hummus

- ¼ medium avocado, diced

- One tablespoon of lime juice

- 3 tablespoons pico de gallo

Instructions

In a bowl, mix the quinoa and the beans. In a tiny bowl, combine the hummus and the juice of one lime, then thin the mixture with water to the desired consistency. Season the beans and quinoa, which drizzle over some of the hummus dressing. Sprinkle with cilantro, pico de gallo, and avocado.

Nutrition Facts

Calories: 500g, Fat:16g, Carbs:74g, Protein:20g

9.3 Roasted Vegetable

Preparation time: 15 Minutes

Making time: 05 Minutes

Servings: 2 Persons

Ingredients

- 1 cup of roasted vegetables from the root family

- 2 tablespoons of olive oil that is extra-virgin

- 1 teaspoon of cumin that has been ground

- 1 teaspoon of ground chili peppers

- 1/2 teaspoon of coriander that has been ground

- Half a teaspoon of kosher salt

- A quarter of a teaspoon of ground pepper

- corn tortillas that have been warmed or toasted gently

- ½ avocado sliced into 8 slices

- 1 lime water, cut into wedges and sliced thinly

- Fresh cilantro and salsa, chopped, to be used as a garnish.

Instructions

In a saucepan, mix the roasted root vegetables with the oil, cumin seeds, chili sauce, and coriander, along with salt and pepper. Cook with the lid on for six to eight minutes over moderately low heat until it is completely cooked through. Spread the mixture on the tortillas in an even layer, with avocado on top. Serve with slices of fresh lime. Depending on your taste, top with chopped cilantro and/or salsa.

Nutrition Facts

Calories: 343g, Fat:17g, Carbs:44g, Protein:3g

9.4 Vegan Cafe Snack Bag

Preparation time: 10 Minutes

Making time: 08 Minutes

Servings: 1 Person

Ingredients

- 1/4 of a cup of hummus

- 1/2 pita bread made with whole wheat, sliced into 4 wedges

- 2 teaspoons mixed olives

- 1/2 English cucumbers, cut into spears

- 1/4 of a big red bell spice, sliced

- 1/4 teaspoon of freshly chopped dill

Instructions

Put the hummus, olives, pita, bell peppers, and cucumber in a resealable container with four cups of space and arrange them. (If you want to keep the spread of hummus and olives apart from each other, you may put them in individual silicone baking mugs before arranging them.) The cucumber should be topped with dill. Freeze until prepared to use and store in an airtight container.

Nutrition Facts

Calories: 194g, Fat:9g, Carbs:23g, Protein:8g

9.5 Collard Greens with Lentils and Apple Slices

Preparation time: 10 Minutes

Making time: 05 Minutes

Servings: 3 Persons

Ingredients

- 1/2 cup of lentils, cooked

- 1 1/2 servings of salad greens

- One apple halves after being cored and sliced

- Vinegar from red wine, 1 tbsp

- 1 1/2 teaspoons of feta cheese, crumbled

- Extra-virgin olive oil, to taste, 2 tablespoons

Instructions

Salad with lentils, roughly half the apple pieces, and feta cheese on top. Toss with oil and vinegar. Accompany with the leftover pieces of apple on the side.

Nutrition Facts

Calories: 347g, Fat:13g, Carbs:48g, Protein:13g

9.6 Use-All-the-Broccoli Stir-Fry

Preparation time: 45 Minutes

Making time: 05 Minutes

Servings: 2 Persons

Ingredients

- 1/2 pounds, with 1-inch-thick stems.

- Large broccoli heads (4-5 total) weighing 2

- 1 red onion, medium

- Shaoxing rice wine, dry sherry, or 2 tbsp.

- 1/2 a cup of water, split

- Two teaspoons of low-sodium tamari

- Toasted Sesame Oil (about 4 tablespoons)

- Splash of chili-garlic paste, 1 tbsp.

- Cornstarch, 2 tablespoons

- Peanut oil equaling 2 teaspoons, divided

- Sugar, Light Brown, 1 Teaspoon

- 1/8 teaspoon

- 1/2 inch fresh ginger, chopped

- Two little red peppers, cut (and seeded, if you want)

- 2 tbsp. of unsalted, roasted peanuts, diced

Instructions

Take broccoli stems and cut off the florets. Separate the florets into pieces of 1 inch in length. Reduce the length of the stems. Spiralize as much from every stem as you may with a vegetable spiralizer fitted with the thin-noodle blade. Slice the remaining stem into pieces about half an inch long. Spiralize an onion by changing it to a thick noodle blade. In a small bowl, combine 1/4 cup fluid, rice vinegar, chile-garlic dressing, two tablespoons of sesame oil, cornstarch, and brown sugar. Put near the range. Over medium heat, warm one tablespoon of peanut oil inside a big, flat-bottom, carbon steel wok. After around 5 minutes of stirring, the broccoli pasta, stem bits, and onion should be soft. Toss the mixture with the two remaining tablespoons of sesame oil and the salt in a large bowl. Toss in the extra tablespoon of peanut oil, the chilies, and the ginger. Prepare for 15 seconds while stirring continuously. After about a minute, add the florets you set aside and cook while tossing until they begin to brown. Cover and continue cooking for another 3 minutes, or until the broccoli florets are soft, using the last 1/4 cup of water. Toss in the sauce you set out and uncover. Keep cooking and stirring for another minute or until the sauce has thickened. Make a pretty presentation by plating the noodle mixture with the cauliflower on top. Sprinkle with peanuts on top.

Nutrition Facts

Calories: 545g, Fat:14g, Carbs:24g, Protein:11g

9.7 Marinated Tofu Salad

Preparation time: 15 Minutes

Making time: 05 Minutes

Servings: 2 Persons

Ingredients

- The juice of 3 lemons, freshly squeezed

- Extra-virgin olive oil, 2 teaspoons

- 1 teaspoon of cumin seed powder

- 1/4 teaspoon pepper

- 1 tsp. of coriander powder

- 1 (large) package (14 oz.) firm tofu, drained and cut into 3/4-inch cubes

- Chopped romaine lettuce equaling 4 cups

- A couple of teaspoons of tahini

- Cucumber, 2 cups worth, peeled, seeded, and chopped

- Tomatoes (two medium plums) Onions (half a cup, coarsely chopped)

Instructions

In a big plastic bag with a zip-top, mix the oil, the juice of one lemon, garlic, coriander, cumin, and salt. Close the bag and give it a little shake to incorporate the tofu. Put in the fridge for at least half an hour and up to two. Bring a big, nonstick pan up to temperature over medium heat. With a slotted spoon, separate the tofu out of the marinade; set the marinade aside in the bag. Tofu should be cooked for 4–5 minutes on the bottom in a skillet. After 4 or 5 minutes, flip and continue cooking until the other side is browned. Reserved marinade; please pour into a big basin. To the mixture, stir in the tahini. Toss the dressing with the lettuce, cucumber, tomato, and onion. Dress the greens with the heated tofu.

Nutrition Facts

Calories: 331g, Fat:26g, Carbs:13g, Protein:13g

9.8 Summer Grilled Vegetables

Preparation time: 25 Minutes

Making time: 45 Minutes

Servings: 2 Persons

Ingredients

- 1/3 cup of fresh mint, chopped

- Parsley, flat-leaf, new, chopped, 1/2 cup

- juice of half a lemon

- 1/2 teaspoon of dried red pepper flakes

- 2 teaspoons of garlic, minced

- Six tablespoons of high-quality olive oil and a quarter of a cup of total

- 1 pound of trimmed asparagus

- Peppers, 2 red, trimmed, seeded, and sliced in half lengthwise

- 3/4 of a teaspoon of ground pepper and 1 teaspoon of salt

- Two zucchinis, cut in half lengthwise

- 1 red onion, sliced in crosswise half-inch pieces

- 2 squash halves (summer)

- 0.5-inch-thick crosswise slices from 1 medium eggplant

Instructions

Bring grill up to temperature (400-450F). Parsley, rosemary, the juice of one lemon, garlic, smashed red pepper, six tablespoons of oil, 1/4 teaspoon salt, and 1/4 teaspoon pepper should all be mixed together in an average-sized bowl. Apply the rest of the 1/4 cup oil to the vegetables (bell peppers, squash, zucchini, onion, eggplant, and asparagus), then season with the additional three-quarters of a teaspoon of salt and half a teaspoon of pepper. Grill rack oiling is recommended (Hint). Arrange the peppers, squash, zucchini, onion, and eggplants on the greased rack and grill, covered, for 3 to 5 minutes on each side or until cooked but still holding their form. The asparagus should be grilled for about 2–3 minutes on each side or until delicate and grill marks form. Gather the grilled veggies and place them on a plate. Top with the parsley-mint dressing and serve.

Nutrition Facts

Calories: 223g, Fat:18g, Carbs:16g, Protein:4g

BOOK 10: Herbal Use for Children

The dose is decreased to make room for the kid's smaller dimensions and greater weight; almost any plant that is healthy for a grownup is healthy for a child. Children tend to have a more delicate constitution; thus, plants with a milder effect are preferable. In general, herbs improve the body's defenses, calm the nerves, and promote the healing processes already present in the body. They need to be the cornerstone of pediatric herbal medicine.

10.1 Herbs and Their Positive Effects on Children

Herbal treatments have many uses and advantages for kids. For instance, ginger has been shown to calm children's queasy tummies. In a moment, we'll get into the specifics of these advantages. Let's start with a broad overview of the advantages.

10.2 Sleep Benefits

Children who have trouble sleeping may find relief with herbal medicines. Among them are:

1)   Catnip

There must be a good reason why cats find catnip so appealing. It aids in a more comfortable night's sleep for animals of all types, as well as easing muscular tension and digestive issues.

2)   Valerian Root

Valerian root, which is among the most well-known all-natural sleep aids, is especially effective for helping youngsters go to sleep and stay asleep.

3)   Chamomile

This plant is not just a sleep aid but also an anti-inflammatory, anti-anxiety, and antioxidant powerhouse.

4)   Passionflower

Naturally occurring GABA, or gamma-aminobutyric, in the brain is increased, leading to calm and less sleeplessness.

10.3 Immune and respiratory system benefits

In some intriguing ways, herbal treatments may assist youngsters with their respiratory and immunological systems. Among the many beneficial plants found in blossoms, herbs, roots, and strawberries are:

1)   Wild Cherry Bark

This has the dual benefits of clearing the airways and reducing muscular cramps.

2)   Elderberry

This may lessen the risk of developing a respiratory infection of the upper respiratory tract and also decrease inflammation in the body.

3)   Oregon Grape Root

This is useful for preventing respiratory infections and treating GERD and similar stomach problems.

4)   Rose Hips Fruit

Vitamin C helps maintain a healthy immune system and is abundant here.

5)   Thyme Leaf

This miraculous plant has many beneficial effects on the respiratory and immunological systems. Asthma, influenza, bronchitis, and those with allergies may find relief by using this.

10.4 Upset Gastrointestinal Benefits

Not only may herbal treatments for children help strengthen their immune systems and improve their quality of sleep, but they are also quite effective in calming upset tummies in both children and adults. Here are some of the most notable advantages of herbal treatments for children:

1)   Peppermint Leaf

Peppermint may help relieve diarrhea and cramping in the upper gastrointestinal tract, as well as reduce bloating and gas in the digestive tract.

2)   Fennel Seed

This helps to improve digestion, decrease gas, bloating, and discomfort, and relaxes your child's digestive tract in general.

3)   Ginger Root

Ginger, as thyme, is one of those herbs that can be used for just about everything. In addition to enhancing digestion and increasing saliva production, it is capable of doing a great deal more.

Conclusion

The practice of using plants as medicine dates back to prehistoric times. Utilizing plants in a therapeutic capacity in order to treat illness and improve one's overall health and well-being are included in this practice. Because some herbs include active (strong) components, it is imperative that they be used with the same degree of extreme care as conventional medicines.

In point of fact, a large number of pharmaceutical treatments are derived from synthetic versions of substances that exist naturally in plants. These molecules may be found in plants. In one instance, the foxglove plant was the source of the drug Digitalis, which is used to treat cardiac conditions. The practice of using plants to cure illness and improve one's overall health and well-being is known as herbal medicine.

Herbs and other pharmaceutical treatments might have negative interactions with one another; therefore, it is important to use caution when combining the two. Always see your primary care physician (PCP) about any concerns you have about your health, and be sure to inform them regarding any herbal medications you are currently taking or are considering taking. Never switch from prescription drugs to herbal remedies without first seeing your primary care physician about the switch.

Made in United States
Troutdale, OR
01/28/2024

17257455R00058